MEDICAL MARIJUANA FOR THE MID-AGED & THE ELDERLY

by

OTHNIEL J. SEIDEN, MD

TABLE OF CONTENTS

FOREWORD

There are numerous books already written on the topic of Medical Marijuana, most of them encyclopedic in size and content. So why am I bothering to write this intentionally small, concise addition to the already growing list of books?

The difference is that this book is aimed specifically at our aging population, many of whom grew up in a time when pot was not the popular and available product that it is today. Some have never tried marijuana and are unfamiliar with it either as a medication or as a recreational drug. Yet, this is the population that might benefit most from the use of medical marijuana. Below is a list of some of the medical conditions that are benefited, and are known to show improvement by the use of medical marijuana. You will note that these are also conditions, which are prevalent among the elderly:

1. Alzheimer's Disease
2. Anorexia
3. AIDS
4. Arthritis
5. Cachexia

6..   Cancer
7.   Crohn's Disease
8.   Epilepsy
9.   Glaucoma
10   HIV
11   Migraine
12   Multiple Sclerosis
13   Nausea
14   Pain
15   Spasticity
16   Wasting Syndrome"
17   PTSD
18   Parkinson's Disease
19   Insomnia
20   Alcoholism
21   Depression
22   Anxiety
23   ALS or Lew Gehrig's Disease
24   Sickle Cell Disease
25   Decompensated Cirrhosis

Each of these medical conditions will be discussed in greater detail along with how medical marijuana might benefit in the treatment and relief of symptoms for each.

The remaining chapters in this book will be aimed at helping the reader to more fully understand the truth about marijuana, the laws around it, it's potential side effects, and the truth and misconceptions surrounding this truly amazing product.

1

History of Marijuana as a Medicine

Cannabis is purported by some to have been used as a medicine for perhaps as long as 10,000 years. For sure, five thousand years ago, in China Emperor Shen Nung prescribed cannabis for beriberi, malaria, rheumatism, constipation, menstrual cramps, and absent-mindedness, among other illnesses. In ancient India, perhaps even earlier, cannabis was used to lower fevers and relieve dysentery, while in ancient Rome the physician Pedacius Dioscorides prescribed cannabis to treat pain of earache and diminished sexual desire.

Over the following centuries the use of marijuana as medication had been well accepted, even for the use in treatment of tumors and a constantly lengthening list of ailments. Its medicinal use spread to Europe and throughout that continent. Eventually it reached Spain and from there spread to the Caribbean islands, and moved on from there to the South American continent, then up into Mexico. From there it reached the United States in the early 1800s.

In 1854, the United States Dispensary said about cannabis and its uses:

The extract of hemp acts as a decided aphrodisiac, increases the appetite, and occasionally induces the cataleptic state. In morbid states it has been found to produce sleep, to allay spasm, to compose nervous inquietude, and to relieve pain. In these respects it resembles opium in its operation; but it differs from that narcotic in not diminishing the appetite, checking the secretions, or constipating the bowels. It is much less certain in its effects; but may sometimes be preferably employed, when its nauseating or constipating effects contraindicate opium. The complaints to which it has been specially recommended are neuralgia, gout, tetanus, hydrophobia, epidemic cholera, convulsions, chorea, hysteria, mental depression, insanity, and uterine hemorrhage. Dr. Alexander Christison, of Edinburgh, has found it to have the property of hastening and increasing the contractions of the uterus in delivery. It acts very quickly, and without anesthetic effect. It appears, however, to exert this influence only in a certain proportion of cases.

* * *

Marijuana's medical uses were expanded and it was available in most pharmacies up until 1937. At that time and through 1938 Marijuana was made illegal in the United States by act of congress in spite of and over the objection of the American Medical Association, which felt its medicinal value for numerous ailments far too beneficial.

Dr. W. C Woodward of the American Medical Association was the only witness to oppose the bill. The legislative activities committee of the AMA wrote to protest the impending legislation:

There is positively no evidence to indicate the abuse of cannabis as a medical agent or to show that its medicinal use is leading to the development of cannabis addiction. Cannabis at the present time is slightly used for medicinal purposes, but it would seem worthwhile to maintain its status as a medicinal agent, There is a possibility that a restudy of the drug by modern means may show other advantages to be derived from its medicinal use.

However, against all the medical advice, and objection the Marijuana Tax Act was approved by congress in 1937 and cannabis preparations were removed from the United States pharmacopoeia in 1941

Also in 1941, the LaGuardia Committee took an in depth look at the marijuana situation in New York and found the claims it that caused crime, violence, insanity, and death were completely unsubstantiated. As regard to medical use, the LaGuardia report said:

"Marijuana has two qualities which suggest it may have useful actions in man. The first is the typical euphoria-producing action, which might be applicable in the treatment of various types of mental depression; the second is the rather unique property which results in stimulation of appetite."

It is of further interesting that the committee did not shrink from commending euphoria itself as having therapeutic potential, and it also noted more than 50 years ago the greatest 1990's use of cannabis as an appetite stimulant for patients with cancer, Aids or Hepatitis C.

The Controlled Substances Act of 1970 placed illicit drugs into one of five schedule categories, and again the decision as to which schedule a drug was put in was not made by medical experts but by the Justice Department, the Attorney General John Mitchell, and the Bureau of Narcotics and Dangerous Drugs, later named the Drug Enforcement Agency, or DEA. Cannabis was placed in schedule I, designated for drugs with a high potential for abuse and of no medical value.

Almost simultaneously, researchers discovered two new medical uses for Cannabis. First was the ability of Cannabis to reduce intraocular pressure, which recommended its use as a treatment for glaucoma. This led to an interesting legal battle. A schoolteacher, Robert Randall, who suffered from glaucoma, was arrested for using marijuana to keep from going blind. He fought his case through the court systems and in 1976 forced the federal government to provide him with cannabis for this treatment purpose, thus becoming the first legal marijuana smoker in the United States since 1937.

The second discovery was the effect marijuana on the side effects of over 40 kinds of chemotherapy used as treatments for cancer. The most toxic and frequent side effect of chemotherapy is violent, and uncontrollable nausea and vomiting often lasting for hours. Often conventional antiemetic treatments didn't help. It was discovered that patients who smoked cannabis before chemotherapy, reported to their doctors that the illegal drug helped them enormously in stopping the vomiting and even making them hungry, appetite loss also being a problem for chemo patients. This successful use of cannabis in cancer chemotherapy led to the development of an expensive synthetic tetrahydrocannabinol named Marinol, and it was rescheduled into Schedule II. However, the cannabis plant and THC extracted from the natural source, remained in Schedule I.

This well proven antiemetic significance of cannabis also led to its use by many AIDS patients. In the mid 1980's, cannabis became useful both as an appetite stimulant against the AIDS wasting syndrome, and as a remedy against the intense nausea often caused by HIV's takeover of the immune system, as well as the toxicity of AZT therapy.

So how does this remarkable plant work to help and benefit so many human afflictions?

To answer this question let's look at the plant and its components.

Cannabis or marijuana refers to the dried flowers, the leaves, the stems, and the seeds of the *cannabis sativa* plant. All of these parts contain the chemical compounds that produce the mind-altering effects that recreational users seek when smoking or ingesting the plant. More importantly they also provide the components with medical benefits. There are at least 60 chemicals known collectively as **cannabinoids.** Different cannabinoids have differing effects in controlling symptoms of the various medical conditions they can benefit. These components are generally divided into one of two categories:

THC. This is the abbreviation for delta-9-tetrahydro-cannabinol. THC is the component mainly responsible for the mind-altering effect of marijuana that recreational users of pot are seeking. However, it also can help treating symptoms such as nausea and vomiting that are associated with a number of medical conditions and treatments such as chemotherapy.

Cannabinol and cannabidiol. These compounds have some of the properties of THC, but cause far less psychoactive effects or the high recreational users seek.

They have most of the medically beneficial characteristics.

Dronabinol is known by its trade name Marinol. We should mention Dronabinol though it is a man-made version of THC available by prescription. It's used to prevent nausea and vomiting after cancer chemotherapy or to increase appetite lost in many diseases or therapies.

When smoked or otherwise ingested, THC and CBD in marijuana attach themselves to two types of receptors on cells in your body.

CB1 is one such cell receptor. These CB1 receptors are found mainly in the brain, especially in those areas that manage body movement, memory, and vomiting. This partly explains why marijuana can affects balance and coordination, and temporarily may impair short-term memory and learning while under its influence. It also explains how it can be useful in treating nausea, pain, and loss of appetite.

CB2 is the other type receptor, which is found in small numbers elsewhere in your body. These are mainly in organs of the immune system, such as your spleen and lymph nodes. Though the function of these receptors is yet not well understood, they may serve as temporary retardants on immune system function.

After you smoke marijuana, its ingredients usually reach their peak levels in your body in a matter of minutes, and the effects can last up to an hour or longer depending on the individual's sensitivity to cannabis and metabolic rate. When orally ingested cannabis can take several hours to reach its peak levels in your body, and the effects may last for several more hours.

The man made prescription drug Dronabinol, which is taken orally as a capsule, usually takes effect in about 30 minutes and may continue to stimulate appetite for more than a day.

Consider the risks

Though a rapidly growing number of doctors and patients recognize that cannabis has many legitimate medical and therapeutic uses the United States government still disagrees. Federal law still recognizes marijuana as a Schedule I drug, classifying it among the most dangerous drugs that have no recognized medical qualities or uses. If you do not live in one of the growing number of states that have made medical marijuana use legal you take a risk using cannabis for any purpose, medical or recreational. If you are discovered by law-enforcement officers, with cannabis in your possession in any form, the penalty can range from a small fine to a lengthy prison sentence.

Using marijuana may pose some health risks, and so you should always discuss its use with your own medical advisor who knows your personal health situation well. There are several possible consequences to consider especially for patients with high risk factors for certain illnesses, or in situations where coordination or reasoning are important, including:

1. Impairment of thinking and problem-solving skills, and memory or reduced balance and coordination. Cannabis should never be used within hours of driving, using dangerous tools.

2. Increased risk of heart attack. There is some evidence that there might be increased risk of heart attack in patients that have high risk factors for heart disease.

3. Heightened risk of chronic cough and respiratory infections

4. Potential for hallucinations especially with high THC varieties.

5. Marijuana smoke contains some of the carcinogenic hydrocarbons found in tobacco smoke. If you have been a chronic smoker it might be wise for you to use orally ingested cannabis or vaporized cannabis.

Talk To Your Health Care Professional About Using Medical Marijuana!

These risks should be taken into account with your physician if you are considering the use of marijuana for medical purposes.

2

MEDICAL CONDITIONS THAT
BENEFIT FROM USE
OF MARIJUANA

There are two major active chemicals in marijuana that appear to have the most medicinal applications. Those are cannabidiol or CBD, which seems to impact the brain while causing a minimal, if any high, and tetrahydrocannabinol or THC, which has pain relieving properties and relieves other stresses, but also does cause temporary mind altering highs.

These same health benefits can in most cases also be gained by taking CBD and THC orally in cannabis containing edibles or Dronabinol, the synthetic form of marijuana.

Let's look at some of these diseases and conditions that are benefitted by medical marijuana use:

1. It can be used in the treatment of Glaucoma.

Marijuana has been used successfully to treat and prevent the eye disease glaucoma, which causes damaging pressure changes within the eye that can damage the optic nerve causing loss of vision. According to the National Eye Institute: marijuana is known to decrease the pressure inside the eye. Studies done in the early 1970s showed that marijuana, when smoked, lowered intraocular pressure in people with normal pressure as well as those with glaucoma. These effects of cannabis have been shown to slow the progression of the disease and preventing blindness.

2. Marijuana may reverse the carcinogenic effects of tobacco and improve lung health.

Marijuana does not impair lung function and can in some instances increase lung capacity according to a study published in Journal of the American Medical Association in January 2012. Researchers while looking for risk factors of heart disease tested the lung function of 5,115 young adults over the course of 20 years. Tobacco smokers lost lung function over time, however pot smokers actually showed a marked increase in lung capacity. It might be that the increased lung capacity was due to taking deep breaths while inhaling the drug rather than a therapeutic chemical in the cannabis.

3. It can control epileptic seizures.

When marijuana extract and synthetic marijuana was given to epileptic rats it rid the rats of the seizures for up to 10 hours. Cannabinoids like the active ingredient in marijuana, THC controls seizures by binding to the brain cells responsible for controlling excitability and regulating relaxation.

Marijuana extract also decreases the symptoms of the severe seizure disorder known as Dravet's Syndrome. A five year old, Charlotte Figi has Dravet's Syndrome, for which her parents are giving her marijuana extract to treat her numerous daily seizures. During his research for the CNN documentary "Weed," Dr Sanjay Gupta interviewed the Figi family, who treats their 5-year-old daughter using a medical marijuana strain high in cannabidiol CDB and low in THC. The child, Charlotte, has Dravet Syndrome, which causes seizures and severe developmental delays.

The medical marijuana treatment has decreased her seizures from 300 a week to just one about every seven days. Now numerous other children in the state of Colorado, where the treatment is legal, are using the same strain of marijuana to treat their seizures. Physicians who recommended this treatment say the cannabidiol interacts with the brain cells to quiet the excessive activity that causes these seizures.

4. Marijuana seems to stop cancer from spreading.

The CBD in cannabis may keep cancer from spreading was what researchers at California Pacific Medical Center in San Francisco reported in 2007. It seems Cannabidiol stops cancer by turning off a gene called Id-1, was reported in the study published in the journal Molecular Cancer. Cancer cells make more copies of this gene than non-cancerous cells, helping them spread throughout the body. Researchers studied breast cancer cells in the lab that had high levels of the Id-1, and treated them with cannabidiol. Following cell cannabidiol treatment they had decreased Id-1 expression and were less aggressive spreaders.

Further evidence of cannabis's affect on cancer is suggested in Sanjay Gupta's CNN special "WEED," mentioning a few studies in the U.S., Spain, and Israel that suggest the compounds in cannabis could even kill cancer cells.

5. Medical Marijuana decreases anxiety.

In 2010, researchers at Harvard Medical School suggested that that some of medical marijuana's benefits in pain and nausea relief, the two main reasons it's often used for the side effects of chemotherapy, may actually be partially due to reduced anxiety, which smoker's note improves their mood and acts as a sedative in low doses.

Beware, however, higher doses may increase anxiety and may cause temporary paranoia.

6. THC slows the progression of Alzheimer's disease.

That marijuana may be able to slow the progression of Alzheimer's disease is suggested in a study led by Kim Janda of the Scripps Research Institute. This 2006 study was published in the journal Molecular Pharmaceutics, and found that THC, in marijuana, slows the formation of amyloid plaques by blocking the enzyme in the brain that makes the amyloid. These plaques are what kill brain cells thus causing Alzheimer's disease.

7. The drug eases the pain of multiple sclerosis.

Marijuana has proven to ease the painful symptoms of multiple sclerosis, a study published in the Canadian Medical Association Journal suggests. Jody Corey-Bloom studied 30 multiple sclerosis patients suffering painful contractions in their muscles. These patient's symptoms didn't respond to other standard treatments, but after smoking marijuana for just a few days they were in considerable less pain. The THC in the cannabis binds to the receptor cells in the nerves and muscles to relieve the pain. The chemical also helps control the severe muscle spasms.

8. Other types of muscle spasms could be helped too.

Other types of muscle spasms also respond to marijuana. In Sanjay Gupta's CNN report he found a teenager who was using medical marijuana to treat diaphragm spasms, which were found to be untreatable by all conventional, and very strong prescription medications. His condition is called myoclonus diaphragmatic flutter, or Leeuwenhoek's Disease, which causes non-stop spasms in the abdominal muscles. These spasms are not only painful, but they interfere dangerously with breathing and speaking. Smoking marijuana calms his attacks almost immediately by calming the muscles of his diaphragm.

9. Medical marijuana dramatically eases side effects from treating hepatitis C while increasing treatment effectiveness.

The treatment for hepatitis C infection is difficult to endure; its harsh negative side effects include extreme fatigue, severe nausea, intense muscle aches, loss of appetite, and depression. Treatment and its side effects lasts for months. Patients are often unable to finish their treatment course because of these side effects.

A 2006 study reported in the European Journal of Gastroenterology and Hepatology stated that 86% of patients using medical cannabis successfully completed their Hepatitis C treatments, while only 29% of non-smokers completed their therapy. Marijuana not only reduced treatment side effects, but also appeared to improve treatment effectiveness. Statistics indicated that 54% of those patients using marijuana in conjunction with therapy got their viral level lower and kept them low, compared to only 8% of nonsmokers.

10. Marijuana can be used to treat inflammatory bowel diseases.

Marijuana appears to benefit Crohn's disease. Crohn's disease is an inflammatory autoimmune bowel disorder that causes pain, vomiting, severe diarrhea, weight loss, and a variety of other symptoms. A recent study in Israel showed that smoking cannabis significantly reduced Crohn's disease symptoms in 10 out of every 11 patients, and actually caused a complete disease remission in five of those patients. It is admittedly a very small study but with stunning results. However, other research has shown similar results. The cannabinoids from marijuana seem to help the bowel to regulate bacteria and intestinal function.

Patients with inflammatory bowel diseases like Crohn's disease and ulcerative colitis benefit by marijuana use, research at University of Nottingham found in 2010. The chemicals in cannabis, the THC, and the cannabidiol CBD interact with cells playing an important role in bowel function and immune system responses. This study was published in the Journal of Pharmacology and Experimental Therapeutics.

11. Cannabis relieves the discomfort of arthritis.

Marijuana relieves pain and reduces inflammation, which helps to relieve pain and discomfort for people with rheumatoid arthritis, researchers announced in 2011. It also promotes sleep, which arthritis pain tends to interrupt. In a study that further supports this, researchers from rheumatology units at numerous hospitals gave their patients Sativex, a cannabinoid-based pain medicine. After just a two-week period, people on Sativex had a significant reduction in pain and much improved sleep compared to patients on placebos.

12. Cannabis helps your sugar metabolism and seems to help keep weight down.

A study published in the American Journal of Medicine suggested that marijuana smokers are skinnier than the average and have healthier metabolism of sugars, this in spit of often eating more calories because of the "munchies" cannabis tends to cause.

This study was of more than 4,500 adult Americans, 579 of who were current marijuana smokers, those who had smoked during the past month. About 2,000 had admitted using marijuana in the past, while 2,000 others in the study had never used the drug. The researchers studied their response to eating sugars, their levels of the hormone insulin, and their blood sugar levels while they hadn't eaten in nine hours, and again after eating sugar. Not only were the marijuana users skinnier, but also they had a healthier response to the ingested sugar.

13. Cannabis improves the symptoms of Lupus.

Medical marijuana is being used to treat the autoimmune disease Systemic Lupus Erythematosis, in which the body starts to attack its own tissues and organs for unknown reasons. The chemicals in marijuana seem to have a soothing effect on the immune system, which is probably how it deals with symptoms of Lupus. Further positive impact of the marijuana is due to its effects on pain and nausea.

14. Marijuana soothes tremors for people with Parkinson's disease.

Research done in Israel shows that smoking marijuana significantly reduces the pain and tremors of Parkinson's disease, and markedly improves the sleep for patients. Above all, most impressive was the improvement of fine motor skills among the patients. Medical marijuana is legal in Israel for many conditions, thus a great amount of valuable research into the medical uses of cannabis is done there, and the research is supported by the Israeli government.

15. Marijuana helps veterans and victims suffering from PTSD.

The Department of Health and Human Services recently signed off on a proposal to allow study of marijuana's potential for treatment for veterans with post-traumatic stress disorder.

Marijuana is already approved to treat PTSD in some states. It is interesting that in New Mexico, PTSD is the number one reason for people getting a medical marijuana license. This is the first time the U.S. government has approved a proposal that incorporates smoked or vaporized marijuana, which is still classified by the government as a drug with no accepted medical applications. Israel again leads in research for the use of PTSD having used it for some time in the treatment of holocaust survivors and their own military veterans. THC appears to help regulate the system that causes fear and anxiety in the body and brain.

16. Marijuana has been shown to protect the brain following a stroke.

Researchers from the University of Nottingham show that cannabis may help protect the brain from damage caused by stroke. Marijuana appears to reduce the size of the area affected by the stroke as shown in rats, mice, and monkeys.

This isn't the only research that has shown the neuro-protective effects of cannabis. Some research shows that the plant may help protect the brain after other traumatic events such as concussions.

There is some evidence that marijuana not only protects the brain, but also can help heal the brain after a concussion or other traumatic injury. A recent study in the journal Cerebral Cortex showed that at least in mice, marijuana lessened the bruising of the brain and helped with healing mechanisms after a traumatic injury. Of great importance to sports medicine, Harvard professor emeritus of psychiatry and marijuana advocate Lester Grinspoon recently wrote an open letter to NFL Commissioner Roger Goodell, saying that the NFL should stop testing players for marijuana, and instead the league should start funding research into cannabis's ability to protect the brain. A growing number of "doctors and researchers believe that marijuana has incredibly powerful neuro-protective properties, an understanding based on both laboratory and clinical data," he writes. In response Goodell recently said that he'd consider permitting athletes to use marijuana if medical research shows that it's an effective neuro-protective agent.

17. Cannabis can help eliminate nightmares.

For people suffering from serious nightmares, especially those associated with PTSD, Cannabis can be helpful. Nightmares and other dreams occur during REM, Rapid Eye Movement stages of sleep. Cannabis tends to interrupt REM sleep, so those dreams may not occur. Research into using a synthetic cannabinoid showed a significant decrease in the number of nightmares in patients with PTSD. Additionally, marijuana may be a better sleep aid for patients than some other substances people use to promote sleep, such as prescription medication and alcohol.

18. Cannabis reduces pain and nausea from chemo, and stimulates appetite.

One of the most recognized medical uses of marijuana is for cancer patients undergoing chemotherapy. Most cancer patients treated with chemo suffer from painful nausea, vomiting, and loss of appetite, which can cause additional health complications. Marijuana can dramatically reduce these side effects by alleviating pain, decreasing nausea, and stimulating the appetite. An increasing number of oncologists are now actively suggesting cannabis in conjunction with chemotherapy.

19. Marijuana can help people trying to cut back on drinking, and other addictions.

It is somewhat ironic that what some people consider to be a gateway drug, marijuana, is actually used by many to curb their addictions. Marijuana is far safer than alcohol; it is much less addictive and doesn't cause nearly as much physical damage to the body and its organs. Research reported in Harm Reduction Journal shows that some people use marijuana as a less harmful substitute for alcohol, prescription drugs, and the illegal drugs. Among of the most common reasons for patients and addicts to make a substitution to cannabis are the less adverse side effects from marijuana and the fact that it is less likely to cause withdrawal problems. You might say it is *a gateway drug to sobriety*. That said, some people may become psychologically dependent on marijuana, and this doesn't mean that it's a total cure for substance abuse problems, however, from a harm-reduction standpoint, it can be very helpful.

20. Marijuana can stimulate creativity and improve activity in the brain.

Marijuana usage has actually been shown to have some positive mental effects, particularly in terms of stimulating and increasing creativity. Although people find that short-term memories tend to function worse when high, people improve their function at tests requiring them to come up with new ideas. One study tested participants on their ability to come up with different words related to a concept, and found that using cannabis people came up with a greater array of related concepts. Cannabis seems to make the brain better at detecting remote associations that lead to radically new ideas.

Other researchers have found that some people improve their verbal fluency, and their ability to come up with different words, while using marijuana. This may help overcome those disturbing *"Senior Moments."* This increase in creative ability and improved brain function may come in part of from the release of dopamine in the brain, lessening inhibitions, and also allowing people to be more relaxed, and giving the brain the ability to perceive things differently.

21. Migraine headaches

Migraine headaches that have not responded to other treatments often respond to cannabis by easing significantly, shortening duration, and in most cases relieving completely. Replacing more addictive prescription medications with medical marijuana is a far better way to treat any chronic or recurring pain.

Many other uses for medical marijuana

The listing above is just a partial inventory of all the medical conditions and situations helped by medical marijuana. In the chapter on the states that allow medical marijuana and the conditions for which it can legally be used in those states, you will see a far greater and amazing listing of its uses.

3

Why You Should Consider Marijuana As a Medication

As of the date of this book's publication 23 of the 50 US states and the District of Columbia, Washington DC, have legalized the medical use of marijuana.

Those who support the use of medical marijuana argue that it is a safe and effective treatment for the symptoms of cancer, AIDS, multiple sclerosis, pain, glaucoma, epilepsy, PTSD, and many other conditions. Their arguments are supported by dozens of research studies carried out by prominent medical organizations, major government reports, and the use of marijuana as medicine throughout the world, and throughout history.

Multitudes of seriously sick and afflicted people, and their doctors, have found medical marijuana to be the only medicine that relieves their pain and suffering, and treats the symptoms of their medical condition, without debilitating side effects of conventional prescription drugs. Medical marijuana has been shown to successfully alleviate the symptoms of a great variety of serious medical conditions, and is often a more effective, and safer alternative to prescription painkillers.

Medical Marijuana Access and Research

Twenty-three states and the District of Columbia have passed medical marijuana laws legalizing the use and production of medical marijuana for qualifying patients under state law. Keep in mind, even in states where medical marijuana laws exist, patients, and providers are vulnerable to arrest and interference from federal law enforcement. However, to date the federal government is not going after legal users, growers, and providers who stay within state marijuana laws. Federal marijuana prohibition has severely prevented cannabis research within the United States, and much of the research carried out has been in more progressive countries like Israel.

As the number of a states passing more liberal medical marijuana laws increases, support for improving existing state medical marijuana programs, and protecting medical marijuana patients, draws nearer. Ending the federal ban on marijuana research within the United States will help more patients have safe access to quality medicine

Mayo Clinic States: When is medical marijuana appropriate?

"Studies report that marijuana has possible benefit for several conditions. State laws vary in which conditions qualify people for treatment with medical marijuana."

Depending on which state you live in, you may qualify for Mayo Clinic treatment with medical marijuana if you meet certain requirements and have one of the following conditions among others:

❖ Multiple sclerosis or severe muscle spasms

❖ Cancer associated with chronic pain, nausea or vomiting, or Severe wasting

❖ Epilepsy or seizures

❖ Glaucoma, although the American Academy of Ophthalmology doesn't yet recommend medical marijuana

❖ Crohn's disease

❖ Terminal illness

❖ HIV/AIDS

❖ Tourette's syndrome

❖ Amyotrophic lateral sclerosis (ALS)

❖ Anorexia

❖ Chronic pain from any condition, though this is a qualifying condition in only a few states

If you are experiencing uncomfortable symptoms or side effects of medical treatment, especially pain and nausea, talk with your doctor about all your options before trying marijuana. Doctors may consider medical marijuana as an option if other treatments haven't helped."

You can use medical marijuana in several forms, including:

- ❖ Oil

- ❖ Pill

- ❖ Vaporized

- ❖ Nasal spray

- ❖ Smoking dried leaves and buds

Certification and use at Mayo Clinics in various states:

Arizona

In Arizona, medical marijuana is legal as plant material to smoke. The Mayo Clinic campus in Arizona does not dispense medical marijuana, certify people for using it, or allow its use on campus or in the hospital.

Florida

In Florida, the state's Department of Health Office of Compassionate Use has not completed rules to allow use of some forms of low-dose medical cannabis under a 2014 law. No smoking of the plant material is authorized. The state's medical cannabis program will be available to people with cancer or other conditions with chronic seizures or severe and persistent muscle spasms.

Georgia

Georgia allows people to be registered in a medical marijuana program by a physician licensed in Georgia. But it has no state-authorized dispensing sites.

Iowa

Iowa allows people to be registered in a medical marijuana program by a physician licensed in Iowa. But it has no state-authorized dispensing sites.

Minnesota

In Minnesota, medical cannabis is available as pills, oils, and liquids at state-designated dispensaries, as of

July 1, 2015. To receive medical cannabis from a dispensary, Minnesota residents with qualifying conditions need to register with the Minnesota Department of Health. As part of the registration process, a physician, physician assistant or advanced practice registered nurse (APRN) must certify that you have a qualifying medical condition.

Mayo Clinic's practices in Minnesota may certify Minnesota residents with qualifying conditions in the Minnesota medical cannabis program. Not all Mayo Clinic health care providers will be registered for the certification process in Minnesota.

Rochester, Minnesota, is the site of one of eight approved medical cannabis-dispensing sites in Minnesota. The others will be in Eagan, Hibbing, Eden Prairie, Minneapolis, Moorhead, St. Cloud, and St. Paul. In Minnesota, marijuana for medical use is not available at pharmacies or through a prescription from a doctor.

Wisconsin

In Wisconsin, marijuana for medical use is not legal.

Is Medical marijuana for you?

The decision as to whether or not you should use medical marijuana is a personal decision that should be made by you and your physician. Though medical marijuana has been found to be safer than many conventional prescription drugs, especially prescription pain meds, which have been shown to be far more addictive, and in some cases has been the only medical intervention to work for certain illnesses, there are some side effects to be considered.

These side effects should be discussed with your physician, who knows your special medical needs and possible risks.

4

Marijuana Delivery Methods

When it comes to medical cannabis consumption, the delivery method is perhaps the next most important consideration. If you find yourself within this category but aspire to become a comprehensive cannabis aficionado, let this be your checklist. Gaining maximum benefits of medical cannabis largely depends on how it's consumed. Each method of consumption provides unique effects.

The three basic delivery methods are inhalation, oral, and topical. Under these three umbrella delivery methods are various sub-techniques, each appropriate for different purposes.

INHALATION DELIVERY METHODS

When marijuana is inhaled, the smoke or vapors enter the lungs to be absorbed into the bloodstream. The two established types of inhalation methods are smoking and vaporization.

Smoking method

This is the most common method of inhalation associated with cannabis. Health professionals are in general agreement that smoke-free methods pose less health risk and are medically preferred.

There are a wide assortment of devices at the smoker's preference, including hand pipes, water pipes, rolling papers, hookahs, and homemade devices.

Hand Pipes

These are probably the most common smoking devices used today and are favored for their convenience. They are small, easily manageable, simple to carry, and use. They function by carrying the smoke created from burning cannabis in their bowls, which is then inhaled by the consumer. Their function is not unlike a tobacco smoker's pipe, though they come in a multitude of designs, very different from tobacco pipes.

Water Pipes

Like hand pipes, water pipes come in a large variety of styles and designs but they are increased in complexity by incorporating water as a filter. The health benefits associated with the addition of water are questionable. Water tends to cool the smoke, but it is debatable if it is really an effective filter for harmful components.

Rolling Papers

Rolling papers are generally used to smoke joints, which are cannabis rolled in a thin paper. Blunts are cannabis rolled in cigar paper actually made from tobacco leaf and thus contain nicotine. Blunt smokers prefer the flavor, smell, and combined effects of the nicotine and cannabis. The added medical risks linked to nicotine and other tobacco carcinogens discourage most health-conscious cannabis consumers.

Hookahs

This is one of the least used methods of smoking cannabis. Cannabis is seldom smoked alone in a hookah because the plant burns faster than it can be inhaled, producing an acrid taste, and too great a wasting of the product, as large quantities of marijuana are needed to yield the same results as other smoking methods. To resolve this economic problem, cannabis is often sandwiched between tobacco, which introduces the same health concerns associated with blunts.

Homemade One-Time Use Devices

This includes all cannabis smoking devices that are homemade or adapted to deliver cannabis smoke to the user. The method allows for the greatest creativity and there is probably no limit to inventions and gadgets used, but the most common homemade device is some form of pipe due to its simplicity.

Vaporization

Vaporization is the logical choice for health-conscious cannabis consumers. A vaporizer heats cannabis to a temperature that is high enough to extract the THC, CBD, and other cannabinoids, but is kept too low to burn the marijuana keeping the potentially harmful toxins that are released in smoke from combustion. In other words, vaporization eliminates the health risks associated with smoking. A side benefit comes with a significant reduction in the cannabis-burning odor. There are an expanding variety of vaporizer types as the technology improves. Many vaporizers take cannabis concentrates, which come in a variety of forms including oil and wax.

ORAL DELIVERY METHODS

Oral delivery includes all products that are administered through the mouth, which include tinctures, ingestible oils, and cannabis infused foods and drinks. Tinctures are essentially a topical application that is administered through the mouth, but they are immediately absorbed into the bloodstream through the oral mucosal membranes, unlike edibles or drinks, which are absorbed in the stomach.

Tinctures

Tinctures are liquid cannabis extracts used by consumers seeking both dosage control and a fast-acting effect, without the health risks associated with smoking. Most commonly, alcohol of proof greater than 80 is used as the solvent, but other fat-soluble liquids can be used as well, such as vinegar or glycerol. Generally, just three or four drops of the tincture are placed under the tongue, where it is directly absorbed into the body instead of being swallowed and digested. When ingested, tinctures are instantly absorbed in an empty stomach but still require time to be processed through the liver, thus reducing dosage control.

Ingestible Oils

Ingestible oils are an in-between method to edibles and tinctures in that they are swallowed and digested like an infused product, but often have the consistency of oil. These oils can either be eaten or put in easily swallowed capsules.

Edibles

Edibles can be defined as any food that contains cannabis. These products have a considerably longer onset and tend to cause more powerful psychoactive effects.

Infused food and drinks can be made a variety of ways, but most often, edibles are infused using an ingredient high in fat such butter or olive oil that enable extraction of the plant's therapeutic properties. Adding tinctures to foods is another option for dosage control and simplicity. Keep in mind that eaten cannabis is absorbed slowly through the stomach, especially after eating other food. People used to smoking cannabis may feel that they haven't had enough orally ingested cannabis after not feeling its effect in a few minutes, and so they take more of the edible, which can lead to overdosing, which can in turn cause a serious high and even hallucinations.

TOPICAL DELIVERY METHODS

Topical cannabis administration utilizes a thick oil extract that has been decarboxylated to activate cannabinoids. Once the cannabinoids are activated, they can be absorbed through your skin.

The topical effects of cannabis differ from other medicating methods in that they do not provide the cerebral stimulation that users describe as being high. Topicals are appropriate for consumers needing a clear head and localized relief such as muscle aches or joint soreness.

5

SIDE EFFECTS AND
WHO SHOULD <u>NOT</u> USE
MARIJUANA

Medicinal marijuana therapy isn't for everyone, and specifically not for you if you have some condition that could get worse with the use of marijuana, in cases where the risks might outweigh the benefits. That's true for any type medical treatment, conventional medical treatments included. Also patient's who have preexisting psychiatric disorders like schizophrenia, or who have a strong family history of mental illness, might have bad reactions to marijuana. That is not to say they shouldn't use medical cannabis, but their private physician or mental health counselor should very carefully monitor them.

Medical cannabis therapy should be absolutely contraindicated for patients who have a severe allergy to the pollen in marijuana or to any of the compounds in marijuana. Also if medical marijuana interferes with some essential other type of therapy that the patient need it should be contraindicated, or overall therapy should be reviewed with the prescribing physician or physicians. In some states transplant candidates awaiting organ transplants, may be disqualified if there is marijuana in their system.

Keep in mind that there remains a conflict here between federal and the state law when it comes to the use of marijuana as a medicine. Presently it is the administration's policy to not interfere with state laws, but if a more conservative administration is elected in the future that may change. If you are made anxious by this risk, though it is not presently great, then use of medical marijuana is probably not right for you at this time. However if you and your medical advisors feel that the benefits to you do indeed outweigh these risks, therapy might be right for you.

Who Should Definitely Avoid Cannabis Use

Healthy Teens

While cannabis consumption is far safer than many things teens will experiment with, there is some evidence that teens who consume cannabis before the age of 16 are susceptible to permanent changes in the brain. Some researchers suggest that heavy use of marijuana before the age of 25 might lead to permanent brain changes or personality changes. More research in this area is needed. However, promising areas for the treatment children and teens with cannabis include treatment of epilepsy, cancer, autism, and other select diseases where cannabis can provide incredible symptomatic relief, and in some cases can markedly alter the disease process. Cannabinoids should also be used cautiously, especially in teens, if there is a family history of psychosis, or if any user is at a high risk of developing psychosis.

Anyone wishing to become pregnant should avoid cannabis.

There is actually little scientific evidence on this subject; however, it is probably wise to err on the side of caution for anyone who wants to conceive. Preliminary research raises the concern that due to the high anti-angiogenic affect of cannabis, which prevents growth of new blood vessels, it is thought that cannabis use could prevent the egg's adhesion to the uterine wall and lead to a miscarriage.

Elderly People

The elderly should keep in mind that cannabis may cause dizziness, or could affect their balance. For this reason they should take all necessary precautions to ensure their safety when using cannabis.

6

WEED IS NO LONGER
A WEED

Marijuana or cannabis has long been lovingly called weed, because it has long been classified as a weed. It, if allowed, will grow like a weed, spread like a weed, and if it grows like a weed, spreads like a weed, it probably is a weed. The only difference is, that unlike a weed, a lot of people want this to grow.

But today's marijuana, at least that cultivated for medical use, can no longer be considered just a weed. The cannabis cultivated for medical use has, in most cases been bred and scientifically altered, and nurtured, and made hybrid, so the plants and their characteristics can actually be categorized by their quality and quantity of medically active components, the THC and CBD.

Some grow operations produce only organic products. Some grow plants that are specially developed to produce the oils that safely treat infants and children with epilepsy and other seizure or neurologic illnesses.

If you go into a medical marijuana dispensary you will be surprised at how knowledgeable the sales people are. If you tell them what your symptoms or medical problems are for which you are seeking relief, they will direct you to the best and most proper varieties of medical cannabis available. There are available high THC brands for patients needing a lift out of depression, high CBD types for pain relief, hybrids with varying combinations of CBD and THC for the treatment of nausea, appetite depression, or appetite enhancement, combinations to produce sleep, while others will cause euphoria and increased activity.

Today's marijuana plant is no longer a weed, but a scientifically developed, cultivated, and nurtured plant with specific qualities categorized into the medical benefits for which it was bred.

7

WHY MARIJUANA WAS MADE ILLEGAL IN THE UNITED STATES

To understand the marijuana laws in the United States today we have to go back to the early 1900's, shortly following the Mexican Revolution, which caused an influx of immigration from Mexico into southern states like Texas and Louisiana. Of course these new immigrants brought with them their native language, culture, and customs, but also the use of marijuana as a medicine and relaxant.

At the time Americans were quite familiar with "cannabis" as a medication since it was present in almost all tinctures and medicines at the time, the word *marijuana* was foreign to them. And to many Americans these new immigrants created fear and bigotry.

Following the fear and bigotry the media began to play on the fears that the public had about these new citizens, spreading false claims about these *troublesome and dangerous Mexicans* with their dodgy native behaviors including the use of marihuana. What the majority of the rest of the nation didn't know was that this marijuana was the same they had in their medicine cabinets.

Actually, the United States Census of 1850 counted 8,327 hemp plantations that were growing cannabis hemp for cloth, canvas, and even the cordage used for baling cotton.

Thus the demonization of the cannabis plant was a natural expansion of the demonization of the Mexican immigrants. In their effort to control of these new immigrants, El Paso, TX did what San Francisco did, to control Chinese immigrants, which was to outlawed opium decades earlier. The idea was to have an excuse to search, detain and deport Mexican immigrants, and like opium to control the Chinese, that excuse was marijuana.

Among the first state laws outlawing marijuana may have been influenced, not only by Mexicans using cannabis, but also because of Mormons using it. Some Mormons who traveled to Mexico in 1910 came back to Salt Lake City with marijuana. The church's reaction to this may have contributed to that state's marijuana laws. Other states quickly followed suit with marijuana prohibition laws, including Wyoming (1915), Texas (1919), Iowa (1923), Nevada (1923), Oregon (1923), Washington (1923), Arkansas (1923), and Nebraska (1927). From bigotry and fear these laws tended to be specifically targeted against the Mexican-American population.

In the eastern states, the "marijuana problem" was attributed to the Latin Americans and black jazz musicians. Marijuana and jazz musicians who used it freely, traveled from New Orleans via Kansas City to Chicago, and then on to Harlem, where marijuana seemed to become a key part of the popular music scene. And again, racism became a major part of the indictment against marijuana. Newspaper editorial columns proclaimed, "Marihuana influences Negroes to look at white people in the eye, step on white men's shadows and look at a white woman twice." An additional fear-tactic, which was spread through the media, that Mexicans, Blacks and other foreigners were introducing white children to marijuana, and marijuana was linking them to violent behavior.

The Federal Approaches to Drug Prohibition

In 1930, a new division in the Treasury Department was established; it was named the Federal Bureau of Narcotics, and Harry J. Anslinger was named its director. This marked the beginning of the federal all-out war against marijuana.

Harry J. Anslinger

Anslinger was an extremely ambitious man, and recognized the Bureau of Narcotics his career opportunity. He saw his new government agency as his chance to define both the problem and the solution. He came to realize that opiates and cocaine weren't problems enough to build him and his agency's importance, so he hit on marijuana to make it illegal at the federal level.

Anslinger immediately turned to the effective themes of racism and violence to draw national attention to the marijuana problem he needed to create. He promoted wild tales of ax murderers on marijuana, and sex, and Mexicans, and Negroes, and foreigners, and violence. Among the quotes he spread that have been attributed to Anslinger and his Gore Files:

"There are 100,000 total marijuana smokers in the US, and most are Negroes, Hispanics, Filipinos, and entertainers. Their satanic music, jazz, and swing, result from marijuana use. This marijuana causes white women to seek sexual relations with Negroes, entertainers, and many others. The primary reason to outlaw marijuana is its effect on the degenerate races.

"Marijuana is an addictive drug which produces in its users insanity, criminality, and death. Reefer makes darkies think they're as good as white men.

"Marijuana leads to pacifism and communist brainwashing.

You smoke a joint and you're likely to kill your brother.

Marijuana is the most violence-causing drug in the history of mankind."

And he used his favorite version of the definition of the word "assassin":

"In the year 1090, there was founded in Persia the religious and military order of the Assassins, whose history is one of cruelty, barbarity, and murder, and for good reason: the members were confirmed users of hashish, or marijuana, and it is from the Arabs' 'hashashin' that we have the English word 'assassin.'"

Self-Serving Yellow Journalism

Harry Anslinger got some additional and timely help from William Randolf Hearst, who owned a chain of newspapers. And Hearst had lots of personal reasons to help Anslinger. Secondly, and probably more important, he was heavily invested in the timber industry to support his newspaper chain, and didn't want to see the development of hemp paper as competition. Thirdly, he had lost 800,000 acres of timberland to Poncho Villa, so he hated Mexicans. And then, telling lurid lies about immigrant Mexicans and the devil marijuana weed drug causing violence sold newspapers, which made him wealthier.

This campaign of bigotry and invented violence became the major force in passing the Marijuana Tax Act of 1937, which effectively banned its possession, use, and sales.

Years later this Act was ruled unconstitutional, so it was replaced with the Controlled Substances Act in the 1970's, which established the Schedules for classifying substances according to their danger and potential for addiction. Cannabis was then placed in the most restrictive category, Schedule I.

Although the Schafer Commission declared that marijuana should not be in Schedule I, and even declined its designation as an illicit substance, President Nixon discounted the report of the commission, and its recommendations, and so marijuana remained, and still remains a Schedule I substance.

Timeline Of Cannabis And Its Legal Standing

1619
Jamestown Colony, Virginia passes a law requiring farmers to grow hemp.

1700s
Hemp was the primary crop grown by George Washington at Mount Vernon, and a secondary crop grown by Thomas Jefferson at Monticello.

1884
Maine becomes the first state to outlaw alcohol.

1906
Pure Food and Drug Act is passed, forming the Food and Drug Administration. This is the first time that drugs have any government oversight.

1913
California, apparently passes the first state marijuana law, it is referred to "preparations of hemp, or loco weed."

1914
Harrison Act is passed, outlawing opiates and cocaine taxing scheme

1915

Utah passes state anti-marijuana law.

1919

18th Amendment to the Constitution calling for alcohol prohibition is ratified

1930

Harry J. Anslinger given control of the new Federal Bureau of Narcotics. He remains in the position until 1962

1933

21st Amendment to the Constitution is ratified, repealing alcohol prohibition

1937

Marijuana Tax Act introduced

1938

Food, Drug and Cosmetic Act introduced

1951

Boggs Amendment to the Harrison Narcotic Act mandatory sentences regarding cannabis

1956

Narcotics Control Act adds more severe penalties for cannabis possession, use, and sales

1970

Comprehensive Drug Abuse Prevention and Control Act.

Replaces and updates all previous laws concerning narcotics and other dangerous drugs. Includes the Controlled Substances Act, where marijuana is classified a Schedule 1 drug, classification reserved for the most dangerous drugs that have no recognized medical use.

8

Is Marijuana a Gateway Drug or Addictive?

Although there are some correlations between marijuana and other addictive drugs, there is no conclusive evidence that one actually causes the other.

The gateway theory refers to the idea that marijuana, in this case, leads its users to eventually abuse other addictive drugs. Though studies of large populations have indeed found that some of those who smoke marijuana are more likely to use other drugs, these studies show a correlation but not causation. The fallacy is, just because marijuana smokers might be more likely to later use cocaine, or some other drug, does not imply that using marijuana causes one to use these other drugs.

A 1999 report from the Institute of Medicine, a branch of the National Academy of Sciences, stated clearly, "In the sense that marijuana use typically precedes rather than follows initiation into the use of other illicit drugs, it is indeed a gateway drug. However, it does not appear to be a gateway drug to the extent that it is the cause or even that it is the most significant predictor of serious drug abuse; that is, care must be taken not to attribute cause to association." The scientific community shares no consensus on the issue of marijuana being a gateway drug, and there is little evidence on the underlying cause and effect.

Social and cultural concerns

The cultural and social concerns pointing to a gateway theory point to the possibility that simply by being around marijuana and the people who use it one might be more likely to end up trying other drugs as well. There is also the suggestion that an individual who uses marijuana may simply be a person more likely to engage in risk-taking behavior, and will seek out and experiment with other drugs. This would suggest there is no causal link from marijuana to other drugs, but rather a social link to people who make it possible to be introduced to other more difficult-to-obtain substances.

An argument for legalizing marijuana is that legal cannabis providers have too much at risk to their licensing to risk selling other illegal drugs, while the street corner illegal provider will try to push the marijuana smoker into more costly, lucrative and addicting drugs. In other words marijuana's illegal status may contribute to its gateway effects by simply introducing smokers to other illegal drugs , which means a marijuana user would be more likely to have access to other illegal drugs through social interactions, and the act of actually buying the drugs illegally.

A *Drug and Alcohol Dependence* study found that marijuana use was far less associated with other illicit drug use in the Netherlands, where marijuana can legally be purchased in so-called coffee shops, than in other countries including the United States.

The fact is that most studies indicate there is no firm ground to stand on when making claims of the marijuana's gateway effect. In fact since medical marijuana is being used successfully to help addicts to get off of alcohol and other addictive illegal and prescription drugs one might say it is a gateway drug to sobriety.

9

HIGH CBD TO LOW THC RATIO STRAINS AND HEMP CBD

Cannabis high CBD strains have become most popular among people who suffer from constant anxiety, stress, and chronic pain. They have found relief with this natural, harmless cannabinoid derived from the same family of plants as medical marijuana. But with all the high CBD strains available today it is becoming far more difficult to find the ideal one for your own purposes because not all CBD strains have the same effects. Each person reacts differently to CBD; some will need high CBD strains to get the results they desire while others can get by with lower strengths.

The five most popular high CBD strains.

#1 ACDC

#2 Cannatonic

#3 Harlequin

#4 Critical Mass

#5 Charlotte's Web

In addition to the most popular and commonly bought CBD strains of medical marijuana, there are many others that might be an even better fit for you. Below, is a listing of 45 other high CBD medical marijuana strains popular among CBD users.

SATIVA STRAINS:
CBD Mango Haze

Mango Haze is a very potent CBD strain having a sweet, peppery flavor suggestive of the tropical mango fruit. Its ratio of CBD to THC is between 2:1 and 1:1, making it ideal for patients who suffer from stress and are wishing to relax without a remarkable high. Still, the effect is quite euphoric, calm state of mind, allowing for completing of simple chores. Mango Haze can aid in patients with lack of appetite and in mild pain.

Charlotte's Web

The best thing about this CBD strain is its very, low less than 0.3% THC content, which makes it the popular choice for use in children suffering from seizures. Charlotte's Web was originally cultivated for a young epileptic patient named Charlotte. The CBD content in this strain is very high, and makes a serum with an earthy/woody taste. It is also used for relaxation and combating mild pain. This strain can cause dizziness and mild anxiety in sensitive users.

Dance World

This CBD strain was cultivated to produce a euphoric, happy state of mind. The CBD content is high and idyllic for those suffering from stress, lack of focus, and diminished energy. Dance World is a hybrid strain made from two other strains, Dancehall and Juanita La Lagrimosa. This gives it an earthy taste with flowery, sweet undertones. This is the preeminent choice for those patients who want an uplifting, pleasant experience without the side effects of a high.

Harlequin

Harlequin is the perfect CBD choice for those wanting to relieve their chronic pain without too much sedation and to avoid the dangerous side effects of prescription painkillers. Harlequin was cultivated by cross breeding four different strains and thus has very strong sativa effects with a dependable 5:2 CBD to THC ratio. This ensures that the users won't face a strong THC high while the CBD produces the pain-relief and anti-inflammatory effects. This strain may bring about dry mouth and eyes in some cases.

Hawaiian Dream

This CBD strain focuses on reducing stress and giving emotional relief to consumers. Hawaiian Dream is the result of the cross breeding of two strains and has a 2:1 CBD to THC ratio, so there is no powerful buzz or debilitating haze, while it still offers a calming effect and clearing of the mind. It is ideal for patients who want to overcome anxiety and still be able to work and be reasonably productive.

Island Sweet Skunk

This CBD strain is mainly used for muscle spasms and anxiety relief. Island Sweet Skunk CBD strain offers relaxation and a clear, calm mind without a strong high. The flavor is quite odd, often described as "skunky," with sweet undertones and a tropical tang. The high CBD content is ideal for stress relief without the highs caused by THC rich strains. Patients will still feel quite energetic and clear-headed though it might cause dry mouth and eyes.

Jamaican Lion

Jamaican Lion is perhaps best for the creative individual who wants a clear, focused mind. Jamaican Lion has an interesting tropical flavor with hints of sage and earthy undertones. This strain is exceptionally good for combating everyday chronic pains. It may cause dry mouth but it leaves the head clear while containing just enough THC to cheer you up.

Johnny's Tonic

Johnny's Tonic is an exceptionally potent and popular CBD strain, which won the cannabis-cup award in 2014 for its high CBD content and promising medical benefits. This is one of the best strains for consumers wishing to combat fatigue, inflammation, stress, and muscle spasms. It has a very pleasant lemon-flowery taste with a skunky undertone. This strain has very low hallucinogenic and paranoia effect while giving clarity and a relaxed state of mind.

CBD MediHaze

This strain is best suited for stress relief and relaxation. A mix of four other strains, to give a great 1:1 CBD to THC ratio, cultivated this high CBD strain. One of the most pleasant things about MediHaze is its intricate aroma and taste reminiscent of mint, spices, and pine. Many describe the flavor as "pleasantly peppery." This strain causes enough of a buzz to induce euphoria but not reaching the "pot-head" level.

Raphael

With a revealing peach flavor and very high CBD to THC ratio, Raphael is the perfect CBD strain for patients who want little to no high but very potent pain relief and a relaxing effect. Raphael can have 1% or less of THC. Likelihood of side effects is very low. Raphael is a perfect choice for patients who are sensitive to THC but still need the beneficial effects of appetite increase, stress reduction, and pain relief.

Swiss Gold

Swiss Gold is a potent sativa CBD strain bred for a 2:1 CBD to THC ratio. Swiss Gold induces a relaxed state that leaves you energized and keeps your awareness sharp. Swiss Gold has a citrusy flavor with earthy undertones, but with a hint of a diesel aroma. It is most often used for headaches, high stress levels, and depression as it is known to increase happiness. It may cause light anxiety and dry eyes in some cases.

HYBRID STRAINS:

ACDC

This hybrid strain is well known for its high CBD to THC ratio. ACDC contains less than 1% THC while packing around 19% potent CBD, meaning that you get a potent relaxing effect without the psychotropic miasma. ACDC has an earthy flavor of citrus with woody undertones. It is usually chosen for pain relief and you get a calming, soothing effect from ACDC. ACDC may sometimes cause dry mouth and dizziness.

Avi

This is a balanced hybrid that is half-sativa and half-indica. Avi is best known for its characteristic berry-like flavor. Delicious and with a 2:1 CBD to THC ratio, this strain is quite potent to increase creativity and energy levels. At this ratio, a mild high is experienced with less of a sedation effect than found in a pure THC experience. There is a chance of having dry eyes and mouth after use; a side effect is quite common in cannabis use.

Avi-Dekel

Avi-Dekel is mainly used to soothe digestive disorders, decrease inflammation, and help patients with sleep disorders. With a high CBD level of almost 16% Avi-Dekel gives you a happy, euphoric experience without the lows associated with a real high. This makes it great for medical use by those not seeking psychoactive effects. Its use may cause dry mouth and mild anxiety in some cases. The taste is earthy with woody and pine undertones. Avi-Dekel is best taken at the end of the day.

Blueberry Essence

With a sweet taste like blueberries, Blueberry Essence offers a calming CBD experience. It is most often chosen by patients seeking to relax into sleep, usually because anxiety, muscle spasms, or pain keeps them awake. While this strain can sometimes cause dry mouth, it is quite popular among patients who experience anxiety attacks and THC highs with regular medicinal cannabis use.

Canna-Tsu

Bred from two high CBD strains, Canna-Tsu offers pain relief and a very relaxing experience. This particular hybrid is well known for its citrusy aroma and earthy tang. Often chosen by patients suffering from anxiety disorders, Canna-Tsu offers a clear-headed high that allows the user to focus on chores and work while relieved from pain and stress. This strain is good for taking in the morning if necessary.

Cannatonic

Cannatonic is a hybrid strain that delivers a CBD to THC ratio of 1:1. It has a quite strong effect compared to others with less THC but gives a lot more clarity than straight marijuana use. The effects are generally calming, with a euphoric feeling and pain relief. It's ideal for patients who want to switch from marijuana to CBD-rich strains. Cannatonic has an earthy flavor reminiscent of pine.

Dieseltonic

This CBD strain is quite potent with a 1:1 CBD to THC ratio. Often chosen for use in mental disorders like depression and anxiety, Dieseltonic gives more mental clarity than typical THC-dominant strains, with better focus and a happy euphoria. The taste is quite different, reminding one of diesel and orange, so be prepared for a unique flavor experience. Dieseltonic may cause dry eyes and mouth.

GI001

GI001 is one of the best high CBD strains if you want lots of benefits but a very low chance of a high. With a ratio CBD to THC of 24:1, GI001 is frequently used for children and adults with epileptic seizures, and patients who get anxiety attacks from high-THC strains. Its pleasant citrus flavor offers a mix of lemon and lime. This is best for patients who want no high, just relief and relaxation.

Harle-Tsu

Ideal for pain relief, Harle-Tsu is a two-strain hybrid that offers a very high CBD to THC ratio of 20:1. It has an earthy flavor with citrusy undertones and a spicy sensation. Patients who want a relaxing experience combined with pain relief, and an uplifting experience like Harle-Tsu. There is little chance of getting a real high, or psychoactive effects. You may experience dry mouth, but this is a common side effect.

Maui Bubble Gift

Maui Bubble Gift is a hybrid of three high CBD strains. Maui Bubble Gift is chosen for its almost double CBD to THC content, which offers a mild, relaxing high with a clearer head. Best used for treating pain, anxiety, and inflammation, some psychoactive effects can be expected, depending on patient sensitivity. With a pleasant flavor reminiscent of berries and woody, earthy undertones, Maui Bubble Gift is the choice of many patients who want to lower their THC intake.

Midnight

This CBD strain was developed to combat nausea and lack of appetite. It's high CBD content helps soothe depression and anxiety, and offers a state of euphoria. It also helps with insomnia and an inability to calm down. With a taste reminiscent of flowers, like lavender and rose, Midnight is quite popular with patients. Use may sometimes cause dry mouth and eyes, but these side effects are quite common in cannabis use.

Nebula II CBD

This is a great choice for patients who need to con-sume medical cannabis, Nebula II has an even 1:1 CBD to THC ratio that offers a mellow high with many of the other benefits of cannabis use. These benefits include pain relief, reduction of inflammation, and the ability to relax into a happy, euphoric state. Nebula II has a sweet, honey-like taste that makes it quite popular. This is an ideal choice for those new to CBD-rich strains.

OG Ringo

OG Ringo is commonly considered a tasty strain that delivers a euphoric, happy high with more mental clarity than do THC-dominant strains. It may cause a spark of creativity and focus in some while combating the symptoms of depression and anxiety. OG Ringo is often chosen for patients with mental illnesses to combat a drop in productivity and happiness.

One to One

This strain offers an average ratio 1:1 of CBD to THC. One to One is a great choice for patients who do not tolerate THC well, who get anxiety attacks from high THC strains, or who simply don't want the side effects of a high. With a citrusy aroma and earthy flavor, One to One offers a highly relaxing yet focused high that doesn't mess with your head or get you too dizzy.

Purple Cheese

With a flavor strongly reminiscent of cheese and blueberries, Purple Cheese has a high CBD content and is favored by patients seeking relaxation. The high and effect might be stronger than in other high CBD strains, so it is best used at night for patients who need to wind down, get rid of bad thoughts, and be able to relax into sleep in a euphoric state. Use may cause dry mouth.

Ringo's Gift

For patients who seek a relaxing, pleasant high without the heaviness and inability to function, Ringo's Gift is an excellent choice. With a 1:1 CBD to THC ratio, this high CBD strain can be too much for those who don't want any high or psychoactive effects at all but is ideal for patients who want a lighter cannabis experience. It's often used for soothing stress and headaches; Ringo's Gift has a pleasant earthy taste and pungent aroma.

Sour Tsunami

Sour Tsunami was one of the first cultivated with the purpose of offering more CBD than THC, even if only by a little. Sour Tsunami offers up to 11% CBD and around 10% THC. The taste is earthy and reminds one of a mix of citrus and pine. This is best chosen by patients wishing to relax and relieve pain without as much of a high.

Trident

The aroma can be quite pungent but is pleasantly sweet and earthy. Trident has a double CBD to THC ratio, which combats pain and stress while offering only a mild, more high. This strain can contain up to 12% CBD, making it one of the really high CBD strains with only around 6% THC. Best used late at night.

Valentine X

Valentine X is able to spark creative thoughts. This CBD strain is very low in THC and offers 25 times as much CBD, making it ideal for combating seizures and epilepsy. It is often chosen for treatment of cancer patients, epileptic children and adults, as well as inflammation. Valentine X has no psychoactive effects. This is why it is chosen by many patients who don't want a high at all, but just health benefits.

VCDC

VCDC was the winner of the 2015 SoCal Medical Cup. VCDC is a potent CBD strain that offers pain relief, relaxation, and increase in appetite, as well as suppressing nausea. VCDC is designed to be good for cancer patients seeking relief from nausea and pain but is also popular for anxiety disorders and for combating stress. VCDC has a very pleasant berry flavor with citrusy hints and an earthy undertone.

Warlock

Warlock is potentially helpful in improving focus and alertness in ADD/ADHD patients. Warlock is also used to induce a calm, alert high in those seeking to relax without inhibiting productivity. The flavor of Warlock is quite earthy with skunky undertones. Best chosen by beginners and patients who want mild effects, it may cause paranoia in some cases.

Zen

With a 1:1 ratio of CBD to THC, Zen is the choice of those patients who want a mild high while retaining clarity. Best used for treating stomachaches, Crohn's Disease, and nausea. Zen helps patients relax, and increase appetite. The taste is earthy with citrus hints and a pungent aroma. There is a chance of getting dry mouth and eyes from Zen, and patients who appreciate a bit of a high prefer it.

INDICA STRAINS

Afghani CBD

With a sweet taste of blueberries, Afghani CBD offers a pleasurable experience. This CBD strain is chosen to combat insomnia and stress, but it can also be quite useful for patients suffering from depression and anxiety disorders. It offers a relaxing high that gently lulls you through a euphoric state and into sleep. It may help stabilize mood in patients with ADD/ADHD.

CBD Shark

With an even THC to CBD ratio, this high CBD strain offers powerful pain relief and relaxation with much less of a high than THC-dominant strains. Patients who don't mind some psychoactive effects but generally appreciate a clearer mind and relief from stress and pain choose it. It is sweet and earthy with a hint of herbs and garlic.

Critical Mass

Critical Mass is a THC-heavy CBD strain with up to 22% THC and is good for strong pain relief and relaxation. It is great for patients who want a strong high with increased CBD their intake. The flavor is citrusy and generally sweet with earthy notes. Use can help soothe the symptoms of insomnia and depression, offering a relaxing, euphoric state. Critical Mass is also good for patients with muscle spasms. It may cause dry eyes and mouth.

Dark Star

Dark Star is known for increasing creativity and a calming high. High in both CBD and THC, Dark Star can have average-intensity psychoactive effects. Dark Star is used for stress and pain relief as well as helping soothe the symptoms of depression and insomnia. With a pungent aroma and woody, earthen undertones, dry mouth or eyes are not uncommon.

Devil Fruit

This high CBD strain is great for muscle spasms and relaxation. Devil Fruit is a strong 70% indica CBD strain that gives patients a mild high with mental clarity. Devil Fruit has a sweet and spicy, woody flavor. Good for combating depression and stress and helping patients to sleep. It has some psychoactive effects, but not as strong as in a higher THC strain. It may cause dry eyes.

Digweed

This CBD strain is best taken at night or when you lie down to rest or nap, as its main effect is to help patients relax and fall asleep. Best chosen to help against insomnia, pain that keeps you awake, and inflammation. Digweed contains enough THC to cause a mild high and should not be taken if you have a productive day ahead of you. Its flavor is sweet with a delicious aroma and woody undertones.

Haoma

Haoma is a CBD strain that's 70% indica and is often chosen to help relieve stress and pain. Haoma is ideal for full-body pain relief without causing too much of a mental high or haziness. The characteristic flowery, sweet taste reminds one of berries and is described as pleasant by most patients who try Haoma. You should take Haoma only before going to sleep and not at the start of a productive day.

Pennywise

Pennywise is often taken for insomnia and depression. Pennywise has an even ratio of CBD to THC making it give a milder high with more mental clarity, but it will still cause sleepiness for most patients. The flavor is spicy and herby with woody undertones. Pennywise is also used to ease symptoms of PTSD, anxiety disorders, and epilepsy. It has a strong relaxing effect and gives a euphoric state.

Remedy

This CBD strain is quite low in THC containing less than 1%, and very high in CBD, containing up to 15%. Remedy allows patients to have a euphoric, calmer state of mind without psychoactive effects. The flavor is sweet, woody, and earthy. It is great for patients who want to soothe pain and stress, and be able to sleep easier without getting high.

Stephen Hawking Kush

This is a low-THC, high CBD strain that helps patients relax and feel happier. It is often used to combat symptoms of depression, fatigue, and chronic pain. Stephen Hawking Kush doesn't cause paranoia or strong psychoactive effects; it simply giving a mellow, euphoric high feeling. The flavor is quite pleasant with hints of lemon, honey, and berry. It may cause dry eyes and dizziness in rare cases.

Sweet and Sour Widow

This is best for patients who suffer from chronic pain and stress. Sweet and Sour Widow offers a mild state of calmness and euphoria without strong psychoactive effects or too much of a high. Great for beginners who don't want to fully experience the heavy feeling of a strong THC high. The flavor is earthy with hints of spicy and herbal tones and a pungent aroma. This is best used before going to bed.

Violator Kush

If patients want a strong couch locking high of THC and a good amount of CBD for the extra pain relief, then Violator Kush is the best strain. It makes patients feel relaxed, sleepy and euphoric, offering relief from pain and stress while also helping them to sleep more easily. The taste is mostly of pine and can be quite flowery and earthy. Don't try this at the start of a productive day.

HEMP OIL CBD

This high CBD product comes from the Agricultural or Industrial Hemp plant. It's ratio CBD to THC is virtually 100% CBD to 0% THC, and since the THC has been almost all bred out of it, this product is legal in all 50 states. It is virtually incapable of causing a high or psychoactive response, however it's CBD effects are fully active. Hemp CBD can be delivered by vaporizer, oil drops, or pills and edibles. The following chapter will introduce you to Hemp CBD in further detail.

10

VERY OLD 'NEW KID ON THE BLOCK' HEMP OIL CBD

There is a very bright future for this 5,000-year-old botanical wonder. The fact that industrial hemp oil CBD has the ability to interact with numerous organ systems in the human body, combined with its safety and exceptionally low toxicity, could make it the upcoming miracle medication.

Industrial hemp and medical marijuana both come from the Cannabis Sativa L. plant, but there is a significant difference.

Agricultural or industrial hemp, often referred to as "hemp stalk," grows differently than the THC-containing cannabis, and looks more like bamboo than the familiar looking pot plant. The more familiar looking THC-producing marijuana plants grow to an average of five feet in height, and for best production are spaced six to eight feet apart. On the other hand, agricultural hemp grows to a height of 10 to 15 feet or taller when ready for harvest, and can be grown three to six inches apart. But most important, agricultural industrial hemp has virtually no potential to produce high-content THC when pollinated by members of their own variety. With proper reproduction the genetics will remain similar with virtually no levels of THC. Because of that fact Hemp oil CBD is legal in all 50 United States. Hemp Oil CBD does not require physician's prescription or state registration for purchase or use.

Cannabidiol or CBD, also referred to as a "phyto-cannabinoid," is a plant derivative that can affect appetite, metabolism, pain sensation, inflammation, thermoregulation, vision, mood, and memory, among other aspects of health and body function.

Differences between marijuana and agricultural hemp

Agricultural or industrial hemp and marijuana come from the same genus of plant designated *cannabis*. The term "genus" refers to a family of plants species and not a single species. In other words this means that there are multiple types of the cannabis plant, all of which are cannabis but each having noteworthy differences. The genus of cannabis is includes three distinct species of the cannabis plant: Cannabis sativa, Cannabis indica, and Cannabis ruderalis.

Cannabis sativa is the most commonly known strain of cannabis. It has been cultivated throughout known history numerous uses, which include the production of seed oil, food, hemp fiber used for clothes, paper, and rope, for medicine, and recreation.

Cannabis ruderalis on the other hand is a species native to Russia and is the hardiest of the three, and is able to withstand far harsher conditions than Cannabis sativa or Cannabis indica, but it is relatively poor in cannabinoids having a lower THC content than either sativa or indica.

Cannabis indica, as its name indicates, was discovered in India and is a cannabis species that is shorter and bushier than sativa. Some scientists doubt the existence of Cannabis indica as a distinct and separate species of cannabis.

In nature, Cannabis ruderalis characteristically has the lowest levels of THC, while Cannabis sativa has a higher level of THC than CBD, and Cannabis indica has a higher level of CBD than THC. That's in nature, however, since man has been cultivating cannabis, especially Cannabis sativa, for thousands of years, the effects of man-made pollination selections have led to several different types of cannabis within the same species. These artificial pollinations have been designer selections were aimed at goals depending on the purpose the cannabis was cultivated for.

Artificial selection

Humans have cultivated cannabis since antiquity, and for a variety of purposes. Through artificial selection, different species of cannabis have different properties; some have been used for medicinal purposes, others as food, and others to create clothes, ropes, and other industrial substances.

Industrial hemp has been produced by strains of Cannabis sativa that have been cultivated to produce very minimal levels of THC, and have been artificially selected and bred to grow taller and sturdier. This has enabled the plant to be used successfully in the production of hemp oil, wax, resin, hemp seed food, animal feed, fuel, cloth, rope, paper, and much more. Industrial hemp is exclusively bred from Cannabis sativa.

Medical marijuana is produced mainly from variants of Cannabis sativa, which have been selectively bred to maximize their varying concentration in cannabinoids. Cannabis ruderalis is almost exclusively grown for medicinal purposes, since it naturally has very small quantities of THC. The major difference then between industrial hemp and medical marijuana is that industrial hemp is exclusively made from Cannabis sativa that was specifically bred to produce the lowest concentrations of THC possible. Industrial hemp always has trace amounts of THC and naturally occurring high amounts of CBD having the highest CBD/THC ratio of all cannabis strains. This means that industrial hemp's chemical profile makes it incapable of inducing intoxicating effects and getting you "high" from ingesting it, thus making it legal in all 50 United States.

Industrial Hemp Dietary Supplements

Industrial hemp is naturally rich in CBD and has only trace amounts of THC; many patients are turning to industrial hemp products as alternatives to medical marijuana. Since medical marijuana is not legal in all the states in the US or in many countries worldwide, products made from industrial hemp can be a safe and legal alternative. Patients can get most of the same beneficial effects of medical marijuana from industrial hemp products, and without getting the high.

Industrial hemp products are safe, are made according to federal standards, and are produced in FDA-registered facilities within the US.

The Many Medical Benefits of CBD

Research is still scratching the surface, but cannabidiol is proving to be immensely beneficial for the treatment of many different ailments and disorders, matching most if not all treated by medical marijuana. Its anticonvulsant benefits for children and adults are getting most of the headlines about CBD oil being available to children suffering from epilepsy, CBD can also treat inflammation, pain, anxiety, many neurodegenerative disorders, PTSD, sleep disorders, arthritis, fibromyalgia, nightmares, to name just a few. It has even been linked to the treatment of cancer, easing its pain, nausea of chemotherapy, and loss of appetite. Some studies suggest that CBD retards the growth of cancer and may even kill cancer cells.

CBD is available as oil and as a pill. CBD oil used to treat intractable epilepsy, for example, is administered a few drops at a time with the help of a dropper. No smoking need be involved, however it can be delivered as a vapor using a small vaporizer little larger than a cigarette holder.

CBD From Medical Marijuana Is Still Illegal In Many States

Though CBD or cannabidiol obtained from industrial hemp is legal and considered a dietary supplement, CBD obtained from marijuana is not. This is, as mentioned before, because CBD from hemp contains virtually no THC while that obtained from medical marijuana may contain large concentrations of THC. In states where it is legal, CBD from medical marijuana is dispensed only to those who are able to get a Dr's prescription.

11

STATES WHERE MEDICAL MARIJUANA IS LEGAL AND THE CONDITIONS FOR WHICH IT IS ALLOWED

Alaska

Qualifying conditions to become a medical marijuana patient in Alaska include:

- ❖ Glaucoma
- ❖ HIV/AIDS
- ❖ Cachexia (wasting syndrome)
- ❖ Pain
- ❖ Nausea
- ❖ Seizures
- ❖ Muscle spasms
- ❖ Multiple sclerosis

For a complete list of qualifying conditions and guidelines, please refer to Alaska's application for medical marijuana registry, or catch up on the latest Alaska cannabis news.

Arizona

Qualifying conditions to become a medical marijuana patient in Arizona include:

❖ Cancer

❖ Glaucoma

❖ HIV/AIDS

❖ Cachexia (wasting syndrome)

❖ Pain

❖ Nausea

❖ Seizures

❖ Muscle spasms

❖ Multiple sclerosis

❖ PTSD

For a complete list of qualifying conditions and guidelines, please refer to the Arizona state legislature concerning medical marijuana, or catch up on the latest Arizona cannabis news.

California

Qualifying conditions to become a medical marijuana patient in California include:

❖ Cancer

❖ Anorexia

❖ AIDS

❖ Chronic pain

❖ Cachexia

❖ Persistent muscle spasms, including those associated with multiple sclerosis

❖ Seizures, including, but not limited to, those associated with epilepsy

❖ Severe nausea

❖ Glaucoma

❖ Arthritis

❖ Migraines

Any other chronic or persistent medical symptom that substantially limits the ability of the person to conduct one or more major life activities (as defined by the Americans with Disabilities Act of 1990) or, if not alleviated, may cause serious harm to the patient's safety or physical or mental health.

For a complete list of qualifying conditions and guidelines, please refer to California Proposition 215, with revised Senate Bill 420, or catch up on the latest California cannabis news.

Colorado

Although Colorado has implemented a legal recreational cannabis market, it still operates medical marijuana dispensaries for valid patients. Colorado medical marijuana patients still pay standard sales tax on cannabis but are exempt from the high excise taxes and additional state taxes collected from recreational cannabis sales.

Qualifying conditions to become a medical marijuana patient in Colorado include:

❖ Cancer

❖ Glaucoma

❖ HIV/AIDS

❖ Cachexia (wasting syndrome)

❖ Persistent muscle spasms

❖ Seizures

❖ Severe nausea

❖ Severe pain

For a complete list of qualifying conditions and guidelines, please refer to Colorado's Debilitating Conditions for Medical Marijuana Use, or catch up on the latest Colorado cannabis news.

Connecticut

Qualifying conditions to become a medical marijuana patient in Connecticut include:

❖ Cancer

❖ Glaucoma

❖ HIV/AIDS

❖ Parkinson's disease

❖ Multiple sclerosis

❖ Damage to the nervous tissue of the spinal cord with objective neurological indication of intractable spasticity

- ❖ Epilepsy
- ❖ Cachexia (wasting syndrome)
- ❖ Wasting syndrome
- ❖ Crohn's disease
- ❖ Post-traumatic stress disorder (PTSD)

For a complete list of qualifying conditions and guide-lines, please refer to Connecticut's medical marijuana qualification requirements, or catch up on the latest Connecticut cannabis news.

Delaware

Qualifying conditions to become a medical marijuana patient in Delaware include:

- ❖ Cancer
- ❖ HIV/AIDS
- ❖ Hepatitis C
- ❖ Lou Gehrig's disease (amyotrophic lateral sclerosis, or ALS)
- ❖ Alzheimer's
- ❖ Post-traumatic stress disorder (PTSD)
- ❖ Cachexia (wasting syndrome)

- ❖ Intractable nausea
- ❖ Seizures
- ❖ Muscle spasms
- ❖ Multiple sclerosis

For a complete list of qualifying conditions and guidelines, please refer to Delaware's medical marijuana program guidelines, or catch up on the latest Delaware cannabis news.

District of Columbia (Washington, D.C.)

Qualifying conditions to become a medical marijuana patient in Washington, D.C. include:

- ❖ HIV/AIDS
- ❖ Cancer
- ❖ Glaucoma
- ❖ Muscle spasms
- ❖ Multiple sclerosis
- ❖ Lou Gehrig's disease (ALS)
- ❖ Cachexia (wasting syndrome)
- ❖ Decompensated cirrhosis
- ❖ Alzheimer's

❖ Seizure disorders

For a complete list of qualifying conditions and guidelines, please refer to the District of Columbia's Medical Marijuana Program Patient FAQ, or catch up on the latest Washington, D.C. cannabis news.

Florida

Florida only allows for the use of cannabis extracts that are low in THC and high in CBD, as well as allowing a legal defense for the use of low THC cannabis for medicinal purposes.

Qualifying conditions to become a medical marijuana patient in Florida include:

❖ Severe, debilitating epileptic conditions

For a complete list of qualifying conditions and guidelines, please refer to the Florida Senate's Bill Analysis, or catch up on the latest Florida cannabis news.

Georgia

Georgia only allows for the use of low THC oil (less than 5% THC by weight).

Qualifying conditions to become a medical marijuana patient in Georgia include:

❖ Cancer

❖ Lou Gehrig's disease (ALS)

❖ Seizure disorders related to diagnosis of epilepsy or trauma-related head injuries

❖ Multiple sclerosis

❖ Crohn's disease

❖ Mitochondrial disease

❖ Parkinson's disease

❖ Sickle cell disease

For a complete list of qualifying conditions and guidelines, please refer to House Bill 1 (Haleigh's Hope Act), or catch up on the latest Georgia cannabis news.

Hawaii

Qualifying conditions to become a medical marijuana patient in Hawaii include:

- ❖ Cancer
- ❖ Glaucoma
- ❖ HIV/AIDS
- ❖ Cachexia (wasting syndrome)
- ❖ Pain
- ❖ Nausea
- ❖ Seizures
- ❖ Muscle spasms
- ❖ Multiple sclerosis

For a complete list of qualifying conditions and guidelines, please refer to Hawaii Senate Bill 862, or catch up on the latest Hawaii cannabis news.

Illinois

Qualifying conditions to become a medical marijuana patient in Illinois include:

- Acquired Immunodeficiency Syndrome (AIDS)
- Alzheimer's disease
- Autism*
- Lou Gehrig's disease (ALS)
- Arnold-Chiari malformation and syringomyelia
- Cachexia (wasting syndrome)
- Cancer
- Causalgia
- Chronic inflammatory demyelinating polyneuropathy
- Chronic post-operative pain*
- Chronic pain due to trauma*
- Chronic Pain Syndrome*
- Crohn's disease
- CRPS (Complex Regional Pain Syndrome Type I)
- CRPS (Complex Regional Pain Syndrome Type II)
- Dystonia
- Fibromyalgia (severe)
- Fibrous dysplasia
- Glaucoma
- Hepatitis C
- Human Immunodeficiency Virus (HIV)

❖ Hydrocephalus

❖ Interstitial cystitis

❖ Intractable pain*

❖ Irritable bowel syndrome*

❖ Lupus

❖ Multiple sclerosis

❖ Muscular dystrophy

❖ Myasthenia gravis

❖ Myoclonus

❖ Nail-patella syndrome

❖ Neurofibromatosis

❖ Osteoarthritis*

❖ Parkinson's disease

❖ Post-concussion syndrome

❖ Post-traumatic stress disorder (PTSD)*

❖ Residual limb pain

❖ Rheumatoid arthritis (RA)

❖ Seizures

❖ Sjogren's syndrome

❖ Spinal cord disease (including but not limited to arach-noiditis, Tarlov cysts, hydromyelia & syringomelia)

❖ Spinal cord injury

❖ Spinocerebellar ataxia (SCA)

❖ Tourette syndrome

❖ Traumatic brain injury (TBI)

Recently recommended qualifying conditions soon to be available for Illinois medical marijuana patients.

For a complete list of qualifying conditions and guidelines, please refer to the Illinois Medical Cannabis Pilot Program's FAQ, or catch up on the latest Illinois cannabis news.

Iowa

Iowa allows for the use of high-CBD cannabis extracts with less than .3% THC.

Qualifying conditions to become a medical marijuana patient in Iowa include:

❖ Intractable epilepsy

For a complete list of guidelines, please refer to Iowa Medical Cannabidiol Act Quick Facts, or catch up on the latest Iowa cannabis news.

Kentucky

Kentucky allows for the use of low-THC cannabis or industrial hemp-derived CBD oil. Only those who are participating in a clinical trial or expanded access program are legally allowed to possess CBD oil.

For more information on accessing CBD in Kentucky, please refer to Senate Bill 124, or catch up on the latest Kentucky cannabis news.

Louisiana

Qualifying conditions to become a medical marijuana patient in Louisiana include:

❖ Symptoms related to cancer

❖ Glaucoma

❖ Spastic quadriplegia

For more information on Louisiana's medical marijuana law, please refer to Senate Bill 143, or catch up on the latest Louisiana cannabis news.

Maine

Qualifying conditions to become a medical marijuana patient in Maine include:

❖ Chronic pain that has not responded to conventional therapy for more than six months

❖ Post-traumatic stress disorder (PTSD)

❖ Lou Gehrig's disease (ALS)

❖ Alzheimer's

❖ Cachexia (wasting syndrome)

❖ Cancer

❖ Crohn's disease

❖ Glaucoma

❖ Hepatitis C (active form)

❖ HIV

❖ Inflammatory bowel disease (IBS)

❖ Seizure disorders

❖ Severe muscle spasms (including multiple sclerosis and other diseases causing severe and persistent muscle spasms)

❖ Severe nausea

For a complete list of qualifying conditions and guidelines, please refer to Maine's medical use of marijuana guidelines, or catch up on the latest Maine cannabis news.

Maryland

Qualifying conditions to become a medical marijuana patient in Maryland include:

- ❖ Cachexia (wasting syndrome)
- ❖ Severe, debilitating, or chronic pain
- ❖ Severe nausea
- ❖ Seizures, including those characteristic of epilepsy
- ❖ Severe and persistent muscle spasms
- ❖ Multiple sclerosis
- ❖ Crohn's disease
- ❖ Alzheimer's
- ❖ Cancer
- ❖ Glaucoma
- ❖ HIV/AIDS
- ❖ Hepatitis C

For a complete list of qualifying conditions and guidelines, please refer to Maryland Senate Bill 757, or catch up on the latest Maryland cannabis news.

Massachusetts

Qualifying conditions to become a medical marijuana patient in Massachusetts include:

❖ Cancer

❖ Glaucoma

❖ AIDS

❖ Hepatitis C

❖ Lou Gehrig's disease (ALS)

❖ Crohn's disease

❖ Parkinson's disease

❖ Multiple sclerosis

For a complete list of qualifying conditions and guidelines, please refer to the Massachusetts medical use of marijuana overview, or catch up on the latest Massachusetts cannabis news.

Michigan

Qualifying conditions to become a medical marijuana patient in Michigan include:

- ❖ Cancer
- ❖ Glaucoma
- ❖ HIV/AIDS
- ❖ Hepatitis C
- ❖ Lou Gehrig's disease (Amyotrophic lateral sclerosis, or ALS)
- ❖ Alzheimer's
- ❖ Nail-patella syndrome
- ❖ Cachexia (wasting disease)
- ❖ Severe and chronic pain
- ❖ Severe nausea
- ❖ Seizures
- ❖ Epilepsy
- ❖ Muscle spasms
- ❖ Multiple sclerosis

For a complete list of qualifying conditions and guidelines, please refer to the Michigan Medical Marihuana Registry Program FAQ, or catch up on the latest Michigan cannabis news.

Minnesota

Minnesota does not allow for smokeable cannabis, only a 30-day supply of oils, edibles, and concentrates. Qualifying conditions to become a medical marijuana patient in Minnesota include:

- ❖ Lou Gehrig's disease (Amyotrophic lateral sclerosis, or ALS)
- ❖ Cancer
- ❖ Cachexia
- ❖ Crohn's disease
- ❖ Glaucoma
- ❖ HIV/AIDS
- ❖ Seizures
- ❖ Severe and persistent muscle spasms
- ❖ Terminal illness
- ❖ Tourette syndrome

For more information, please visit the Minnesota Department of Health - Medical Cannabis, or catch up on the latest Minnesota cannabis news.

Mississippi

Mississippi allows access to CBD oil only. Qualifying conditions to become a medical marijuana patient in Mississippi include:

❖ Debilitating epileptic seizure disorders

Patients must receive medical recommendations by a physician from the University of Mississippi Medical Center to participate in the clinical trial. For more information, please refer to House Bill 1231 or Harper Grace's Law, or catch up on the latest Mississippi cannabis news.

Missouri

Missouri allows access to CBD oil only. Qualifying conditions to become a medical marijuana patient in Missouri include:

❖ Intractable epilepsy

For more information, please refer to House Bill 2238, or catch up on the latest Missouri cannabis news.

Montana

Qualifying conditions to become a medical marijuana patient in Montana include:

- ❖ Cancer
- ❖ Glaucoma
- ❖ HIV/AIDS
- ❖ Cachexia (wasting syndrome)
- ❖ Chronic pain
- ❖ Intractable nausea or vomiting
- ❖ Epilepsy or an intractable seizure disorder
- ❖ Multiple sclerosis
- ❖ Crohn's disease
- ❖ Painful peripheral neuropathy

A central nervous system disorder resulting in chronic, painful spasticity or muscle spasms.

For a complete list of qualifying conditions and guidelines, please refer to Montana Code Annotated 2013, or catch up on the latest Montana cannabis news.

Nevada

Qualifying conditions to become a medical marijuana patient in Nevada include:

- ❖ AIDS
- ❖ Cancer
- ❖ Glaucoma
- ❖ Condition or treatment for a medical condition that produces cachexia (general physical wasting and malnutrition)
- ❖ Persistent muscle spasms (including multiple sclerosis)
- ❖ Seizures (including epilepsy)
- ❖ Severe nausea
- ❖ Severe pain

For a complete list of qualifying conditions and guidelines, please refer to the Nevada Medical Marijuana Program, or catch up on the latest Nevada cannabis news.

New Hampshire

Qualifying conditions to become a medical marijuana patient in New Hampshire include:

- ❖ A chronic or terminal disease

❖ Cachexia (wasting syndrome)

❖ Severe pain

❖ Severe nausea/vomiting

❖ Seizures

❖ Severe, persistent muscle spasms

For a complete list of qualifying conditions and guidelines, please refer to New Hampshire House Bill 573, or catch up on the latest New Hampshire cannabis news.

New Jersey

Qualifying conditions to become a medical marijuana patient in New Jersey include:

❖ Lou Gehrig's disease (amyotrophic lateral sclerosis, or ALS)

❖ Multiple sclerosis

❖ Terminal cancer

❖ Muscular dystrophy

❖ Inflammatory bowel disease (IBS)

❖ Crohn's disease

❖ Terminal illness if the physician has determined a prognosis of less than 12 months of life

❖ Seizure disorder, including epilepsy

❖ Intractable skeletal muscular spasticity

❖ Glaucoma

❖ HIV/AIDS

❖ Cancer

For a complete list of qualifying conditions and guidelines, please refer to the New Jersey Medicinal Marijuana Program, or catch up on the latest New Jersey cannabis news.

New Mexico

Qualifying conditions to become a medical marijuana patient in New Mexico include:

❖ Severe chronic pain

❖ Painful peripheral neuropathy

❖ Intractable nausea/vomiting

❖ Severe anorexia

❖ Cachexia (wasting syndrome)

❖ Hepatitis C infection currently receiving antiviral treatment

❖ Crohn's disease

❖ Post-traumatic stress disorder (PTSD)

❖ Lou Gehrig's disease (amyotrophic lateral sclerosis, or ALS)

❖ Cancer

❖ Glaucoma

❖ Multiple sclerosis

❖ Damage to the nervous tissue of the spinal cord with intractable spasticity

❖ Epilepsy

❖ HIV/AIDS

❖ Inflammatory autoimmune-mediated arthritis

❖ Hospice patients

For a complete list of qualifying conditions and guidelines, please refer to the New Mexico Medical Cannabis Program FAQ, or catch up on the latest New Mexico cannabis news.

New York

Qualifying conditions to become a medical marijuana patient in New York include:

- ❖ Cancer

- ❖ Epilepsy

- ❖ HIV/AIDS

- ❖ Huntington's disease

- ❖ Inflammatory Bowel Disease (IBS)

- ❖ Lou Gehrig's disease (ALS)

- ❖ Parkinson's disease

- ❖ Multiple sclerosis (MS)

- ❖ Neuropathies

- ❖ Spinal cord damage

For a complete list of qualifying conditions and guidelines, please refer to the New York State Medical Marijuana Program FAQ, or catch up on the latest New York cannabis news.

North Carolina

North Carolina allows for the use of CBD oil only. Qualifying conditions to become a medical marijuana patient in North Carolina include:

- ❖ Intractable epilepsy

For more information, please refer to House Bill 1220, or catch up on the latest North Carolina cannabis news.

Oklahoma

Oklahoma allows for the use of CBD oil only. Qualifying conditions to become a medical marijuana patient in Oklahoma include:

Must be under the age of 18 suffering from:

❖ Lennox-Gastaut syndrome

❖ Dravet syndrome

❖ Severe myoclonic epilepsy of infancy

❖ Any form of refractory epilepsy not treatable by traditional medical therapies

For more information, please refer to Katie and Cayman's Law (House Bill 2154), or catch up on the latest Oklahoma cannabis news.

Oregon

Qualifying conditions to become a medical marijuana patient in Oregon include:

- Cancer
- Glaucoma
- Alzheimer's
- HIV/AIDS
- Cachexia (wasting syndrome)
- Severe pain
- Severe nausea
- Seizures, including but not limited to seizures caused by epilepsy
- Persistent muscle spasms
- Multiple sclerosis

For a complete list of qualifying conditions and guidelines, please refer to the Oregon Medical Marijuana Act, or catch up on the latest Oregon cannabis news.

Rhode Island

Qualifying conditions to become a medical marijuana patient in Rhode Island include:

- Cancer
- Glaucoma

- ❖ HIV/AIDS
- ❖ Hepatitis C
- ❖ Cachexia (wasting syndrome)
- ❖ Chronic pain
- ❖ Severe nausea
- ❖ Seizures, including but not limited to those characteristic of epilepsy
- ❖ Severe and persistent muscle spasms
- ❖ Multiple sclerosis
- ❖ Crohn's disease
- ❖ Alzheimer's

For a complete list of qualifying conditions and guidelines, please refer to Rhode Island's medical marijuana approved qualifying debilitating medical conditions, or catch up on the latest Rhode Island cannabis news.

South Carolina

South Carolina allows for the use of CBD oil only. Qualifying conditions to become a medical marijuana patient in South Carolina include:

Certain forms of epilepsy as part of a state-run clinical trial.

For more information, please refer to the Medical Cannabis Therapeutic Treatment Research Act, or catch up on the latest South Carolina cannabis news.

Tennessee

Tennessee allows for the use of CBD oil only. Qualifying conditions to become a medical marijuana patient in Tennessee include:

❖ Intractable seizures (as part of a clinical research study).

For more information, please refer to Senate Bill 280, or catch up on the latest Tennessee cannabis news.

Texas

Texas allows for the use of CBD oil only. Qualifying conditions to become a medical marijuana patient in Texas include:

❖ Intractable epilepsy

For more information, please refer to Senate Bill 339, or catch up on the latest Texas cannabis news.

Utah

Utah allows for the use of CBD oil only. Qualifying conditions to become a medical marijuana patient in Utah include:

❖ Intractable epilepsy

For more information, please refer to House Bill 105, or catch up on the latest Utah cannabis news.

Vermont

Qualifying conditions to become a medical marijuana patient in Vermont include:

❖ Cancer

❖ AIDS/HIV

❖ Multiple sclerosis

❖ Cachexia (wasting syndrome)

❖ Severe pain

❖ Nausea

❖ Seizures

For a complete list of qualifying conditions and guidelines, please refer to the Vermont patient marijuana registry FAQ, or catch up on the latest Vermont cannabis news.

Washington

Changes to Washington state's marijuana laws via Senate Bill 5052 will result in the state's medical marijuana industry being absorbed by its recreational cannabis market. These changes will go into full effect July 1, 2016. Until then, medical marijuana dispensaries will still be operational but are ultimately expected to close or incorporate themselves into an existing licensed retail cannabis shop.

Qualifying conditions to become a medical marijuana patient in Washington include:

❖ Cancer

❖ HIV/AIDS

❖ Multiple sclerosis

❖ Epilepsy or other seizure disorder

❖ Spasticity disorders

❖ Intractable pain

❖ Glaucoma

❖ Crohn's disease

❖ Hepatitis C

Diseases, including anorexia, which result in nausea, vomiting, wasting, appetite loss, cramping, seizures, muscle spasms, or spasticity

For a complete list of qualifying conditions and guidelines, please refer to the Washington state legislature regarding medical cannabis, or catch up on the latest Washington state cannabis news.

Wisconsin

Wisconsin allows for the use of non-psychoactive CBD oil only. Qualifying conditions to become a medical marijuana patient in Wisconsin include:

❖ Seizure disorders

For more information, please refer to Lydia's Law (Act 267), or catch up on the latest Wisconsin cannabis news.

Wyoming

Wyoming allows for the use of CBD oil only. Qualifying conditions include:

❖ Intractable epilepsy

For more information, please refer to House Bill 32, or catch up on the latest Wyoming cannabis news.

12

MARIJUANA RESEARCH

Cannabis has been cultivated and consumed by humans since the beginning of recorded history. Cannabis-based textiles dating to 7,000 B.C.E have been recovered in China, and the plant's use as a medicinal and mood altering agent date back almost just as far.

Though one of the anti-cannabis proponents main arguments to change of the drug's schedule 1 status is, " there is too little research of marijuana's medical value," cannabis is in fact one of the most investigated therapeutically active substances in history. There are to date approximately 22,000 published studies or reviews in the scientific literature referencing the cannabis plant and its cannabinoids. Nearly half of these scientific studies and reviews were published within the past ten years according to a key word search on PubMed Central, the US government repository for peer-reviewed scientific research. The scientific conclusions of this research conflicts directly with the federal government's stance that states cannabis is a highly dangerous substance worthy of criminalization.

A February 2010 investigators at the University of California Center for Medicinal Cannabis Research announced the findings of a series of randomized, place-bo-controlled clinical trials on the medical value of inhaled cannabis. The studies, which utilized the 'gold standard' for FDA clinical trial design, concluded that marijuana ought to be a "first line treatment" for patients with neuropathy and other serious illnesses.

Several other studies conducted by the Center assessed smoked cannabis's capacity to alleviate neuro-pathic pain, an extremely difficult to treat type of nerve pain associated with cancer, diabetes, HIV/AIDS, spinal cord injury and many other debilitating conditions. Each of the trials found that cannabis consistently reduced patients' pain levels to a degree that was as high-quality, or better than currently available medications, many of which were far more addicting.

Another study conducted by the same Center's investigators assessed the use of marijuana treatment for patients suffering from multiple sclerosis. The study found that cannabis was superior to placebo in reducing spasticity and pain in MS patients, and provided some benefit beyond commonly prescribed treatments.

The summary of the Center's clinical trials was published in 2012 in the *Open Neurology Journal*, and concluded, "The classification of marijuana as a Schedule I drug as well as the continuing controversy as to whether or not cannabis is of medical value are obstacles to medical progress in this area. Based on evidence currently available the Schedule I classification is not tenable; it is not accurate that cannabis has no medical value, or that information on safety is lacking."

Similarly controlled trials are taking place around the world. A 2010 review by researchers in Germany reports that, "Since 2005 there have been 37 controlled studies assessing the safety and efficacy of marijuana and its naturally occurring compounds in a total of 2,563 subjects." Many FDA-approved drugs go through far fewer trials involving far fewer subjects, according to a 2014 review paper published in the *Journal of the American Medical Association*, "The median number of pivotal trials performed prior to FDA drug approval is no more than two and over one-third of newly approved pharmaceuticals are brought to market on the basis of only a single pivotal trial."

Research in the 1970s, 80s, and 90s primarily assessed cannabis' ability to alleviate disease symptoms, such as nausea associated with cancer chemotherapy; while scientists today are exploring the potential role of cannabinoids to actually modify diseases. For example, scientists are investigating cannabinoids' ability to moderate autoimmune disorders such as multiple sclerosis, rheumatoid arthritis, and inflammatory bowel disease; also marijuana's role in the treatment of neurological disorders such as Alzheimer's disease and amyotrophic lateral sclerosis or Lou Gehrig's disease, and Parkinson's disease. In 2009, the American Medical Association (AMA) urged "that marijuana's status as a federal Schedule I controlled substance be reviewed with the goal of facilitating the conduct of clinical research and development of cannabinoid-based medicines."

Of great interest, researchers are also studying the anti-cancer activities of cannabis, as there appears to be a growing body of preclinical and clinical data, which concludes that cannabinoids can reduce the spread of specific cancer cells via programmed cell death, and by the inhibition of angiogenesis or the formation of new blood vessels.

Israel's cannabis research programs far exceed US research. With over 20 research initiatives underway, they are hoping to validate new alternative patient therapies and to advance the science of cannabis.

Completed Research

Overcoming the Bell-Shaped Dose-Response of Cannabidiol by **Using Cannabis Extract Enriched in Cannabidiol.**

Cannabidiol (CBD), a major constituent of Cannabis, has been shown to be a powerful anti-inflammatory and anti-anxiety drug. However, a bell-shaped dose-response was observed, which limits its clinical use. In the present study, In stark contrast to purified CBD, the clone 202 (Avidekel) extract, provided a clear correlation between the anti-inflammatory and anti-nociceptive responses and the dose, with increasing responses upon increasing doses, making this plant medicine ideal for clinical uses.

Head Researcher: Dr R. Gallily. Zhannah Yekhtin, Lumír Ondřej Hanuš.

Location: The Lautenberg Center for General and Tumor Immunology, The Hadassah Medical School, The Hebrew University of Jerusalem, Jerusalem, Israel.

Published in: Scientific Research Vol. 6 No.2, February 2015

Cannabis Induces a Clinical Response in Patients with Crohn's Disease: a Prospective Placebo-Controlled Study.

Clinical research study that was conducted to examine whether or not cannabis brings about clinical and bio-chemical improvement in cases of active Crohn's disease, without the use of steroids.

Head Researcher: Dr. Timna Naftali.

Location: Gastroenterology Hospital: Meir Medical Center, Kfar Saba, Israel.

Published in: Clinical Gastroenterology and Hepatology, Volume 11, Issue 10, Pages 1276-1280.e1, October 2013.

The Effects of Cannabis on Appetite and Blood Indices of Geriatric Patients

A long-term observational follow-up conducted to collect data from elderly nursing home patients that regularly use medical cannabis. The study measures parameters such as: nutritional blood work, caloric intake, weight, prescription drug usage, sepsis, trembling, spasticity, and quality of life measurements (mood, sleeping habits, etc.)

Head Researcher: Dr. Moshe Geitzen, Geriatrics

Location: Hadarim Nursing Home, Kibbutz Naan

Status: The results of the first two years of the follow-up were presented at two geriatrics conferences and very well received. The follow-up has been extended for a third year based on the positive feedback from the geriatrics research community.

Treatment of Crohn's Disease with Cannabis: An Observational Study

The retrospective research study was conducted by interviewing 20 patients suffering from Crohn's disease that were granted a license for medical cannabis treatment to measure the effectiveness of the treatment. The study has found very positive effects on the symptoms of the disease (number of bowel movements, quality of bowel activity, blood in stool samples, pain, etc.)

Head Researcher: Dr. Timna Naftali, Gastroenterology

Location: Meir Medical Center, Kfar Saba, Israel.

Published in: IMAJ – The Israel Medical Association Journal, Volume 13, Pages 455-458, August 2011.

The prescription of medical cannabis by a transitional pain service to wean a patient with complex pain from opioid use following liver transplantation: a case report.

The purpose of this case report is to describe a patient with a preoperative complex pain syndrome who underwent liver transplantation and was able to reduce his opioid consumption significantly following the initiation of treatment with medical cannabis.

Research in Progress

Effects of Cannabis on Cancer

Conducted by Professor Amos Toren, Head of Pediatric Hemato-Oncology at the Sheba Medical Center – Tel Hashomer using the varieties: Avidekel and Midnight. The study commenced in December 2013 and will carry on through to May 2015.

Effects of Cannabis on Hypokinetic and Hyperkinetic Movement Disorders (Parkinson's)

Conducted by Dr. Tanya Gurevich at Tel Aviv Sourasky Medical Center. The study commenced in February 2011 and will carry on through to May 2015.

Effects of Cannabis On Children With Cancer

Conducted by Professor Amos Toren, Head of Pediatric Hemato-Oncology at the Sheba Medical Center – Tel Hashomer. The study commenced in January 2014 and will carry on through June 2015.

Effects of Cannabis on Tinnitus

Conducted by Dr. Yahav Oron, Otolaryngology, Head and Neck Surgery at the Wolfson Medical Center using the variety: Midnight. The study commenced on November 2013 and will carry on through to June 2015.

Effects of Cannabis on Colitis

Conducted by Dr. Timna Naftali at the Meir Medical Center using the variety: Erez. The study commenced in July 2010 and will carry on through to December 2015.

Effects of Cannabis on Crohn's Disease

Conducted by Dr. Timna Naftali at the Meir Medical Center using the variety: Avidekel. The study commenced in October 2013 and will carry on through to June 2016.

Research Commencing Shortly

Cannabis and IBD Data Collection

Conducted by Dr. Timna Naftali at the Meir Medical Center.

The Effects of Cannabis on Patients with Hepatitis B and C Related Liver Diseases

A study that examines the effects of cannabis on patients with liver diseases related to Hepatitis B and C. The research will be conducted at the Ziv Medical Center in Israel.

The Effects of Cannabis on Dystonia and Spasticity of Cerebral Palsy Pediatric Patients

This clinical trial will examine the effects of cannabis on dystonia and spasticity in children with neurological diseases. The clinical trial will consist of 40 patients divided into four groups which will be administered either a 6:1 or a 20:1 ratio CBD-THC oil. The study will be carried out at the Wolfson Medical Center in Israel.

The Effects of Cannabis on Encephalopathic Epilepsy and Dravet Syndrome in Pediatric Patients

A clinical trial is intended to examine the effects of Avidekel enriched with pure CBD on children with encephalopathic epilepsy. This study will include medical and research teams form 4 different hospitals in Israel.

The Effects of Cannabis on Geriatric Patients Suffering from Dementia-related Restlessness

The study will focus on the effectiveness and safety of cannabis for geriatric patients with Dementia-related behavioral problems and restlessness. Research will be carried out at the Geriatrics Department of the Sanz Medical Center (Laniado Hospital) in Israel.

The above research information From MedRelief.com

THE SAFETY PROFILE OF MEDICAL CANNABIS

Cannabinoids possess a remarkable safety record when compared to other therapeutically active substances, and above all prescription drugs. Studies have shown that the consumption of marijuana, regardless of its quantity or potency, cannot induce a fatal overdose. In fact according to a 1995 review prepared for the **World Health Organization,** "There are no recorded cases of overdose fatalities attributed to cannabis, and the estimated lethal dose for humans extrapolated from animal studies is so high that it cannot be achieved by users."

That said, we must reiterate, ***cannabis should not be viewed as a totally harmless substance.*** Its active constituents may produce a variety of undesirable physiological and euphoric effects. Thus there may be some patients or recreational users that are susceptible to increased risks from the use of cannabis, such as adolescents, pregnant or nursing mothers, and patients who have a family history of psychiatric illness. Also patients with a history of heart disease or stroke may also be at a greater risk of experiencing adverse side effects from marijuana. Cannabis use in and patients prone to falling or dizziness with posture change should take extra precaution while using marijuana.

As with any medication, patients should consult thoroughly with their physician before deciding whether the medical use of cannabis is safe and appropriate.

REFERENCES AND RESOURCES

CNN Weed 3: The Marijuana Revolution - CNN.com

www.cnn.com/specials/health/medical-marijuana

CNN
Explore the latest news on medical **marijuana**. ... Dr. Sanjay Gupta puts medical **marijuana** under the microscope again. "High Profits," a **CNN** ...

Medical marijuana refugees -   Gupta: 'I am doubling down' - Obama backs pot ...

CNN
Sanjay Gupta: Time for a medical marijuana ... - CNN.com
http://www.cnn.com/2013/08/09/health/gupta-weed-reaction

CNN
Apr 20, 2015 - Dr. Sanjay Gupta puts medical **marijuana** under the microscope again with " **Weed** 3: The **Marijuana** Revolution" at 9 p.m. ET Monday on **CNN**, ...

High Profits - CNN.com
www.**cnn**.com/shows/high-profits

CNN

A young couple with a dream seek to build the world's first legal **marijuana** empire. #HighProfits.

CNN Weed 3 Documentary 2015 - YouTube

https://www.youtube.com/watch?v=QnVHxOPEbqc

Dr Sanjay Gupta docu-series on **cannabis**. ... **Weed** HD **CNN Special** Dr Sanjay Gupta 2013 Documentary ...

Dr Sanjay Gupta's CNN Special "WEED" - YouTube

https://www.youtube.com/watch?v=Z3IMfIQ_K6U

Aug 11, 2013 - Uploaded by ThePutipato

Dr. Sanjay Gupta's epic change of heart regarding medical **cannabis** is a momentous occasion for all of us ...

Watch: Jon Stewart mocks CNN's 'High Profits,' 'Weed 3'

Apr 23, 2015 - Of **course** Jon Stewart had some 4/20 fun at the expense of one of the ... Watch: Jon Stewart rips **CNN's** 'High Profits,' '**Weed** 3' — then he gets ripped ... The **special** segment (embedded below): "Uncle Jonny's Super Kush, ...

Here's an anti-legalization group's response to CNN's 'Weed 3'

Apr 20, 2015 - **CNN's** third "**Weed**" documentary debuted Sunday night, and the **program** is **CNN** chief medical correspondent Dr. Sanjay Gupta's biggest ...

CNN 'Weed' Documentary Follows Sanjay Gupta's Reversal ...

Aug 11, 2013 - A remarkable documentary aired on Sunday night on **marijuana**, not necessarily for its conclusions, but for where it ran: **CNN**. The network's ...

WEED 3: The Marijuana Revolution on CNN with Dr. Sanjay ...

Multidisciplinary Association for Psychedelic Studies

... with a **special** focus on MAPS and Dr. Sue Sisley's work to study medical **marijuana** ... Plan to watch the premiere of **Weed** 3 on **CNN** with Dr. Sanjay Gupta on ... These efforts include our lawsuits against the DEA regarding the **application** of ...

Weed Part 1 - CNN - CannabisTube

www.**cannabis**tube.net/video/466/**weed**-part-1-**cnn**

Description: **CNN** medical reporter Dr. Sanjay Gupta researches **marijuana** as a safe, effective drug for seizures, pain management, cancer treatment, and more.

Medical Marijuana - Master Reference From the Shaffer Library of Drug Policy

http://www.druglibrary.org/schaffer

Note: This page was prepared for the November, 1996 election. Some of the external links may be out of date.

In support of the Californians for Compassionate Use initiative and as a resource to all who are interested in the medical marijuana issue, we have established this unified page of medical marijuana resources on the Internet. If you are aware of any research on medical marijuana - pro, con, or indifferent - which is on the Internet but not listed here, please send an e-mail to: cliff_schaffer@yahoo.com

References marked with are the references which we feel are most important to understanding the medical marijuana issue.

Do you think the media ought to know about this page? See our **Media Contact Lists**, for the names and addresses of newspapers, television, and radio stations in your area. Write them a letter today.

My Question:

In all my study and review of the information regarding this issue, one question keeps coming back to me. Let's assume - for the sake of argument - that marijuana has no medical value whatsoever, despite the fact that it has a several thousand year history of medical use and that a prescription drug is made from its primary active ingredient. Let's assume - for the sake of argument - that all these medical marijuana patients are just fooling themselves.

Even in that case, what would we stand to gain as a society by punishing sick people and putting them through an already overloaded criminal justice system? Even if they are deluding themselves — **what benefit is there to prosecuting sick people?**

Cannabis Research Library - A collection of medical research on cannabis

From Cliff Schaffer's site:

Historical Information

In order to properly understand the current medical marijuana issue, it is really necessary to understand the surprising history of marijuana and how the marijuana laws came to be. We recommend the following texts:

From the **Report of the National Commission on Marihuana and Drug Abuse**, 1972

History of the Medical Use What you didn't know about the medical uses will probably surprise you.

History of the Non-Medical Use of Drugs in the United States - by Professor Charles Whitebread. This is a fascinating and highly entertaining 20-page summary of the history of the marijuana laws in the United States. Transcribed from a speech by Professor Whitebread before the 1995 California Judges Conference.

The Forbidden Fruit and the Tree of Knowledge: An Inquiry into the Legal History of American Marihuana Prohibition by Professors Richard J. Bonnie & Charles H. Whitebread, II, Virginia Law Review, Volume 56, October 1970 Number 6 — This is the major research work from which Professor Whitebread drew the information for his speech above.

The British Pharmaceutical Codex, 1934 - relating to cannabis:

For further background information, please refer to:

Major Studies of Drugs and Drug Policy of the last 100 years.

Historical References on Drugs and Drug Policy

Historical information on Hemp/Marijuana
The Marihuana Tax Act of 1937 - **Transcripts of Congressional Hearings and related documents**

MEDICAL INFORMATION
Marijuana as Medicine - Assessing the Science Base - Full text of the report by the National Academy of Sciences Institute of Medicine, 1999.
State Statutes Recognizing Marijuana's Medical Value

Statement of the American Public Health Association in favor of Medical Marijuana

Cannabis Therapeutic Research Program - Report to the California Legislature, Prepared by the Research Advisory Panel - 1989 — The full text of the results of the State of California's investigation into the medical uses of marijuana.

A Critical Review of the Research Literature Concerning Some Biological and Psychological Effects of Cannabis by Dr. Peter L. Nelson (1993). A critical review of the research literature concerning some biological and psychological effects of cannabis. In Advisory Committee on Illicit Drugs (Eds.), Cannabis and the law in Queensland: A discussion paper (pp. 113-152). Brisbane: Criminal Justice Commission of Queensland.

Cannabis Amotivational Syndrome and Personality Trait Absorption: A Review and Reconceptualization by Peter L. Nelson, Ph.D.

Personality Trait Absorption: An Exploratory Study of Opportunity and Capacity in Relation to Cannabis Use by Peter L. Nelson, Ph.D.

Pharmacological Reviews of Marijuana — by Leo E. Hollister, MD Veterans Administration Medical Center and Stanford University School of Medicine, Palo Alto, California from PHARMACOLOGICAL REVIEWS Copyright c 1986 by The American Society for Pharmacology and Experimental Therapeutics

Marijuana and Immunity - by Leo E. Hollister, MD — Journal of Psychoactive Drugs p159-163 Vol.24 Apr-Jun 1992

Medical Uses of Illicit Drugs by Lester Grinspoon and James B. Bakalar

Plaintiff's Reply Brief — Ralph Seeley's successful lawsuit for his own medical marijuana.

Senate Joint Resolution No. 8 - The resolution which passed the California legislature in 1993, calling for the medical use of marijuana. This resolution was vetoed by Governor Pete Wilson because he says that allowing sick people to have medicine "sends the wrong message".

Marijuana as Antiemetic Medicine: A Survey of Oncologists' Experiences and Attitudes by Richard Doblin and Mark A. R. Kleiman

Psychiatric Aspects of Marijuana Intoxication — Samuel Allentuck, MD, and Karl Bowman, MD

Therapeutic Application of Marijuana - Dr. Robert Walton.

An Incident in Kansas - A tale of the harassment meted out to a 100 percent legal medical marijuana user.

The health and psychological consequences of cannabis use - National Drug Strategy Monograph Series No. 25 - By the Australian Government

Marinol Facts — The pharmaceutical facts about Marinol.

Breckenridge, Colorado endorses medical marijuana

Frisco, Colorado endorses medical marijuana

Santa Cruz County Measure A Marijuana For Medical Use Initiative -This measure was passed by over 75% of the vote.

Sonoma County Approves Medical Marijuana

Marijuana Smoking as Medicine, A Cruel Hoax by Gabriel G. Nahas, M.D. and Nicholas A. Pace, M.D.

Marihuana as Medicine: A Plea for Reconsideration by Lester Grinspoon, MD James B. Bakalar, JD Journal of the American medical Association, June, 1995

Marijuana Compassion Clubs by Tim Whitmire Associated Press, August 10, 1995

Information for Physicians — Nausea and vomiting - from CancerNet from the National Cancer Institute's PDQ System — Contains a discussion of nausea and marijuana.

References on Multiple Sclerosis and Marijuana

Editorial from USA Today supporting medical marijuana 7-18-96

Articles by Tod Mikuriya, MD

Tod Mikuriya, MD, is a psychiatrist and Former Director of Marijuana Research for the National Institute of Mental Health

Introduction from Marijuana: Medical Papers by Todd Mikuriya, M.D.

Cannabis as an Adjunctive Treatment for AIDS Related Illness. — By Tod Mikuriya, M.D.

Cannabis as an Adjunctive Treatment for AIDS Related Illness. Part 2 By Tod Mikuriya, M.D.

Possible Therapeutic Cannabis Applications for Psychiatric Disorders by Tod H. Mikuriya, M.D.

Safe Use of Cannabis by Tod H. Mikuriya, M.D.

Consuming Cannabis Safely by Tod H. Mikuriya, M.D.

Medicinal Uses of Hemp Drugs - by Tod Mikuriya, M.D.,

Marijuana Medical Handbook by Tod Mikuriya, M.D.

Marijuana Addicts Anonymous by Lance B., submitted by Tod Mikuriya, M.D.

Marinol and Cannabis by Tod H. Mikuriya, M.D.

Chronic Migraine Headache: five cases successfully treated with

Marinol and/or illicit cannabis. By Tod H. Mikuriya, M.D.

Cannabis and Marinol in the treatment of Migraine Headache by Tod H. Mikuriya, M.D.

Toxic Effects of Marijuana by Tod H. Mikuriya, M.D.

For New Users of Cannabis: The Reynolds Protocol:

Cannabis Medicinal Uses at a "Buyers" Club by Mikuriya, T.H.

Songs by Tod Mikuriya (At least he has a sense of humor!)

Vaporization of Cannabinoids: a Preferable Drug Delivery Route by Tod H. Mikuriya, M.D.

Cannabis 1988 Old Drug, New Dangers, The Potency Debate, Journal of Psychoactive Drugs, Vol 20(1), Jan-Mar, 1988 pg 47. Mikuriya, Tod H. and Aldrich, Michael.

This is a summary of an article discussing the myth of the increase in marijuana potency over the last couple of decades. As this article and others have pointed out, the strongest forms of marijuana have been available since the dawn of recorded history. Readers are invited to make reference to the various historical documents below regarding the historical use of hashish.

ANSWERS TO FREQUENTLY ASKED QUESTIONS ABOUT MARIJUANA USE

This is an excellent summary of many of the questions regarding marijuana. It is very well-documented. Contributed by Christopher Reeve.

The Myth of Marijuana's Gateway Effect by John P. Morgan, M.D. and Lynn Zimmer, Ph.D. This is a good review of the myth that marijuana leads to harder drugs.

PHARMACOLOGY OF MARIJUANA: JUST ANOTHER SEDATIVE by Frederick H. Meyers, M.D., Professor of Pharmacology, University of California, San Francisco, Ca.

A Review of the Scientific Literature Re Amotivational Syndrome
This is an excellent synopsis of the information regarding the "amotivational syndrome" and marijuana. Complete with citations for further reference. Contributed by Brian of DRCNet.

Notes on Marijuana and the Amotivational Syndrome

The human toxicity of marijuana: a critique of a review by Nahas and Latour. This is an abstract of an article which reviewed the work of Dr. Gabriel Nahas regarding his claims about the dangers of marijuana.

Marijuana and the Human Brain - By John Gettman, with NORML

The Effects of Marijuana on Consciousness — From: Altered States of Consciousness, edited by Charles T. Tart, Doubleday & Co., 1972, Chapter 22

Cannabis: the brain's other supplier by Rosie Mestel - reprinted from the New Scientist 31 July 1993 This is an article about natural chemicals in the brain which are very closely related to THC.

Chemical Constituents of Cannabis - Report of a Study by a Committee of the INSTITUTE OF MEDICINE, National Academy Press, Washington, DC 1982

From **Carl Olsen's site**:

DEA Judge Francis L. Young's ruling (September 6, 1988) on Medical Marijuana - The ruling of the Chief Administrative Law Judge of the DEA after hearing two years of testimony pro and con on the issue of medical use of marijuana. **A must read**.

1997 Iowa Legislative Survey

Iowans for Medical Marijuana

The Alliance for Cannabis Therapeutics

Patients Out of Time - Marijuana as Medicine

Jenks v. State, 582 So.2d 676 (Florida, June 13, 1991)

CBS Sixty Minutes ("Smoking to Live") (December 1, 1991)

Declaration of Dr. Daniel Spyker, Food and Drug Admin. (June 16, 1993)

National Center for Toxicological Research - Arkansas Times (September 16, 1993)

National Center for Toxicological Research - Published Journal Articles

Nat'l Institute on Drug Abuse (NIDA) rejects AIDS/marijuana study (April 19, 1995)
AIDS researcher, Dr. Donald Abrams, is critical of NIDA ruling (April 28, 1995)

San Jose Mercury News (May 14, 1995)

Journal of the American Medical Association (June 21, 1995)

Nat'l Institute on Drug Abuse Anti-Marijuana Conference (July 18, 1995)

Ralph Seeley v. The State of Washington (August 25, 1995)

New England Jounal of Medicine (Sept. 7, 1995)

American Public Health Association (November 1995)

H.R. 2618 - therapeutic use of marijuana (Nov. 10, 1995)

The Lancet (November 11, 1995)

The Boston Globe - Pot, a balm to some, faces new hurdle (Nov. 25, 1995)

Potential medical uses of Cannabis, by David W. Pate (December 1995)

State of Washington funds medical marijuana study (March 8, 1996)

Cannabidiol: The Wonder Drug of the 21st Century? (May 25, 1996)

From the MAPS Site:

The following are new as of September 6, 1995.

Dr. Donald Abrams' FDA-approved research protocol (IND#43,542) comparing the effectiveness of smoked marijuana and the oral THC capsule in promoting weight gain in patients suffering from the AIDS wasting syndrome.

Letter to the New England Journal of Medicine

The following are new as of August 11, 1995.

NIDA Rejection Letter from Dr. Leshner Re: Medical Marijuana

Reply to Dr. Leshner by Dr. Donald Abrams

Comment by Rick Doblin on Dr. Leshner's decision

From the Lindesmith Center Site

The Medical Marijuana Issue Among PWAS: Reports of Therapeutic Use and Attitudes Toward Legal Reform by Wesner, Ben. Working Paper No. 3, Working Paper Series, Drug Research Unit, Social Science Research Institute, University of Hawaii at Minoa. June, 1996.

Marihuana as Medicine: A Plea for Reconsideration by Grinspoon, Lester, and James B. Bakalar. Editorial. Journal of the American Medical Association 273.23 (1995): 1875-76.

Therapeutic Potential and Medical Uses of Marijuana by Mikuriya, Tod.

The History of Cannabis by Grinspoon, Lester, and James B. Bakalar in Marihuana: The Forbidden Medicine. [chapter 1] New Haven: Yale University Press, 1993.

Club Medicine by Christie, Jim. Reason, April, 1996:54-57.

Out of Joint: The Case for Medicinal Marijuana by Hecht, Brian. The New Republic. 15 July 1991: 7-10.

From the AIDS Treatment News Archive

04/03/92 - Anti-Drug Politics Impede Medical Use of Marijuana

07/27/91 - Marijuana: Therapeutic Access Threatened

12/01/95 - California: Medical Marijuana Petition Drive Begins

08/07/92 - Medical Marijuana: Overwhelming Support at San Francisco Hearing

01/07/94 - Medical Marijuana: National Press Coverage, No News

12/01/95 - Medical Marijuana: 80% U.S. Voter Support

11/22/91 - Therapeutic Marijuana Initiative Approved by San Francisco Voters

08/05/94 - Medical Marijuana: 89 Percent Support

10/06/95 - California: Marijuana Compassionate Use Statewide Initiative

09/02/94 - California AIDS Legislation — Action Alerts

06/16/95 - San Francisco: Medical Marijuana on Viacom Cable, June 20

08/05/94 - Interim AIDS Coordinator Announced

08/05/94 - Kaposi's Sarcoma — Major Overview Published

09/29/95 - Drug Policy Reform: Ninth International Conference,

October 18-21

12/23/91 - Announcements

10/20/89 - SAN FRANCISCO: AIDS ISSUES ON NOVEMBER BALLOT

From the **High Times site:**

The High Times Medical Marijuana Page

Mississipi and Colorado Nurses Associations Pass Medical Marijuana Resolutions by Al Byrne

The Battle for Medical Marijuana by Peter Gorman

Medical Marijuana Update 10-11-95 by Leslie Stackel

Medical Marijuana Bust May Spur Legal Challenge by Paul Derienzo

Marinol - The Little Synthetic That Couldn't by Elsa Scott

From HempBC (Hemp British Columbia)

Dutch Deport Medical Marijuana User

San Diego Medical Marijuana Activist Arrested In Ohio

From the DRCNet Site

Mother of Two Convicted for Medical Marijuana

A Medical Marijuana Victory - Ralph Seeley

From The Drug Watch International Site:

Just so you won't think that we have restricted this list just to the links which favor medical marijuana, here is some stuff about marijuana from the opposition. We invite you to compare their claims with the research on the other sites.

Marijuana (in general)

Drug Watch International's position paper on "Medical Marijuana" use.

Gabriel Nahas' paper on Hemp, Marijuana and the Law

"Marijuana as Medicine Refuted by NIH Scientists". Dr. Janet Lapey reports on recent findings from the National Institutes of Health. Published in the Best of IDEA, Illinois. Fall, 1993.

This article published in the Best of IDEA shows that no credible organization has supported Medical Marijuana use.

"Marijuana for AIDS Patients?...Think Again." From Drug Watch Oregon.

"GLAUCOMA. Is Marijuana a Safe and Effective Treatment?" From Drug Watch Oregon.

Marijuana Research Review. Volume 1, No.1 February, 1994. A publication of Drug Watch Oregon.

Marijuana Research Review. Volume 1, No.2 July, 1994. A publication of Drug Watch Oregon.
Marijuana Research Review. Volume 1, No.3 October, 1994. A publication of Drug Watch Oregon.

Marijuana Research Review. Volume 2, No.1 January, 1995. A publication of Drug Watch Oregon.

Marijuana Research Review. Volume 2, No.2 March, 1995. A publication of Drug Watch Oregon.

Marijuana Research Review. Volume 2, No.3 June, 1995. A publication of Drug Watch Oregon.

Marijuana Research Review. Volume 2, No.4 September, 1995. A publication of Drug Watch Oregon.

Susan Kaplin's paper on research used to block the UK "Royal Commission on Cannabis" May, 1994.

"MARIJUANA IS NOT MEDICINE. SOMEBODY HAD BETTER TELL YOUR DOCTOR!" by Dan Brookoff, M.D., Ph.D. This **must read** article gives the hard facts about medical marijuana use and enlightens readers about why some Harvard Medical School professors may have come out in favor of it.

"Mental fuzziness linked to marijuana", the Chicago Tribune reports.

The "shadow pushers" are the aging marijuana users and advocates who try to legitimize their drug of choice and perpetuate their crusade to legalize marijuana. They have embraced slick marketing and promotional techniques that target a new generation of potential marijuana advocates. A paper by Rosanna Creighton.

From the Massachusetts Cannabis Reform Coalition, Inc

Federal Medical Marijuana Attracts Bi-Partisan Support; First Two Republicans Sign On To Bill — NORML News Service Story

Massachusetts Medical Marijuana Legislation Progresses - 1-96

From Cures Not Wars

NYC Medical Marijuana Buyers Club Prosecuted by D.A.

Support the new Medical Marijuana Bill in Congress - HR 2618

From the The Scientist - U. of Pennsylvania

Trials Of Marijuana's Medical Potential Languish As Government Just Says No by Peter Gwynne

Links to other sources of information

George McMahon, One of eight patients in the federal medical marijuana program

NORML of Canada Medical Marijuana Page

How to Use Medical Marijuana - From the Orange County Buyer's Club

Ron Shaw's Home Page - A Medical Marijuana User

Marijuana Policy Project
From the Shaffer Library of Drug Policy

http://www.druglibrary.org/schaffer

OTHER BOOKS BY OTHNIEL J. SEIDEN, MD

Health

5 HTP The Serotonin Connection:

The Natural Supplement that helps
you be in control of your mind and body!

ISBN: 1519148445

5-HTP and Depression Management:

Available in Kindle Only

5HTP and Memory Loss Management with:

Available in Kindle Only

5 HTP PMS and Menopause:

Available in Kindle Only

Coping with Arthritis:

ISBN: 151941353X

Coping with BPH:

Benign Prostatic Hypertrophy
Male, over 45, you probably have it!

Available in Kindle Only

Coping with Colorectal Cancer:

Prevention and Cure of theSecond Leading
Cause of Cancer Deaths

Available in Kindle Only

Coping with Fibromyalgia:

It's not in your head, it's a disease!

ISBN: 1519438311

Coping with Prostate Cancer:

Prevention and Cure

of Man's Most Common Cancer

ISBN: 1519438737

Heart of a Woman:

Prevetion and Cure of the #1 Killer in Women

ISBN: 1519441533

Heavy and Healthy:

Forget Your Weight and Get Fit!

ISBN: 1519495412

Quit Smoking Now!:

The Program to Help You

Quit Smoking Now and Forever!

ISBN: 1519495781

Sharpening the Aging Mind:

Methods, Tricks & Tips to

Keep Your Mind Super Sharp

ISBN: 1519496028

Sleep Disorders Management:

Available in Kindle Only

The Second half begins at 50:

Your Longevity Handbook

ISBN: 1519496389

Walk!:

Walk Your Way to Great Health & Long Life

Available in Kindle Only

Weight & Appetite Management:

Available in Kindle Only

Relationships:

Adultery Case Histories:
Why People Cheat on Their Partners
Available in Kindle Only

Communing with the Dead:
Death Needn't Part You
ISBN: 1519190085

Foreplay:
The True Focus of Great Sex
ISBN: 1519440979

Sex in the Golden Years:
The Best Sex Ever, Stay Sexually Active for Life
ISBN: 1519495927

The Big O:
Male & Female Multiple Orgasms
ISBN: 1519496109

The Hospice Experience:
Making Your Most Important Final Decision
ISBN: 1519496281

When Your Spouse Dies:
A widow's & widower's handbook
ISBN: 151949646X

Jewish Fiction

Padre Pio:

The Capuchin – the life of Padre Pio -
St. Pio of Pietrelcina

ISBN: 1519495684

Seed of Avraham:

A 4000 Year History of the Jewish Family...

ISBN: 1519495811

Shtetl:

The Story of a Life No More...
As told from the hereafter

ISBN: 1519496036

The Cartographer:

1492

ISBN: 151949615X

The Condemned Voyage:

The S.S. St. Louis - 1939

Available in Kindle Only

The Crusades:

The Jewish World of the 12th Century

Available in Kindle Only

The Death of Berlin:

A Story of Hollocaust Survival and Revenge

Available in Kindle Only

The Remnant:

The Jewish Resistance in WWII

ISBN: 1519496346

The Uprising of Babi Yar:
The Syrets Deathcamp
Available in Kindle Only

Miscellaneous

Guaranteed Routes to Success for Writers:
A Road Map Through Today's
Dramatic Changes in Publishing
Available in Kindle Only

Joy of Volunteering:
Working and Surviving in Developing Countries
ISBN: 1519495587

So You Want to Write a Book:
ISBN: 1519496079

ABOUT
OTHNIEL J. SEIDEN, MD

Having my professional background in medicine, I learned early on from my patients that one of their biggest complaints was they had difficulty understanding what their doctors and nurses were trying to tell them. This encouraged me to write medical self help book which translated medical and scientific language into easily read and understood lay language. As I have aged my non-fiction has gone more and more to illnesses and sexual matters that face Baby Boomers and Senior Citizens.

LET US KNOW WHAT YOU THINK!

PLEASE LEAVE A REVIEW ON AMAZON.COM

www.ingramcontent.com/pod-product-compliance
Lightning Source LLC
Chambersburg PA
CBHW070242190526
45169CB00001B/268